# Unequal Lives

Health and Socio-economic
Inequalities

# Unequal Lives

## Health and Socio-economic Inequalities

*Hilary Graham*

 McGraw Hill

Open University Press

Open University Press
McGraw-Hill Education
McGraw-Hill House
Shoppenhangers Road
Maidenhead
Berkshire
England
SL6 2QL

email: enquiries@openup.co.uk
world wide web: www.openup.co.uk

and Two Penn Plaza, New York, NY 10121-2289, USA

First published 2007
Reprinted 2010, 2011

A catalogue record of this book is available from the British Library

ISBN-13 978 0 335 22261 2 (pb)  0 978 335 22262 9 (hb)
ISBN-10 0 335 22261 2 (pb)  0 335 22262 9 (hb)

Library of Congress Cataloging-in-Publication Data
CIP data applied for

Typeset by RefineCatch Limited, Bungay, Suffolk
Printed in UK by Ashford Colour Press Ltd, Gosport, Hampshire

The **McGraw·Hill** Companies

For Fiona Raitt

# Contents

# Acknowledgements

This book draws on rich seams of research on social and health inequalities. I have mined these seams in order to build a deeper understanding of the connections between socio-economic inequalities in people's lives and in their health. Certainly there are gaps in research, and important ones which need urgently to be filled. But there is much which is already known, knowledge grounded in studies of a quality that has impressed me deeply. My first debt is to the community of social and health researchers from whom I have learned so much.

Within this community are researchers whose wisdom has been imparted not only through scientific papers and books but through conversations, often continuing over many years. Among this group, I would like to record my gratitude to colleagues in the Economic and Social Research Council (ESRC) Health Variations Programme and the life course group of the European Science Foundation (ESF) Social Variations in Health Expectancy Program for their intellectual generosity. I would particularly like to thank Clare Farquhar and Chris Power for discussions which opened up avenues of analysis which I have continued in this book.

Many others have helped me track down data and advised me on sources of evidence, so willingly and often at very short notice. They include Jonathan Bradshaw, Carol Emslie, Bob Erens, Alissa Goodman, Clare Griffiths, Seeromanie Harding, Juliet Harman, Hazel Inskip, Catherine Law, Barbara Maughan, Tim Mulgan, Lucinda Platt, Steve Platt, Nigel Rice, Sally Stephenson, Carol Thomas, Ian Watt and Margaret Whitehead.

I am grateful to Sue Mendus and Chris Power for comments on Chapter 1 and Chapter 10 respectively, and to Carrie Graham and Carol Smart for feedback and support at all stages of the long writing process. My greatest thanks are reserved for Fiona Raitt who made it all possible.

# Introduction

This book is about people's unequal lives. It is about inequalities in people's lives in two senses. One concern is with inequalities in life and death: with the fact that some people have a better chance of living a long and healthy life than others. Its second concern is with inequalities in the lives people lead: in the social advantages some enjoy and the disadvantages others endure. A central message of the book is that these two aspects of people's unequal lives are two sides of the same coin. Inequalities in people's health are intimately and inextricably connected to inequalities in their material and social circumstances. To understand and confront health inequalities, we therefore need to understand and confront social inequalities.

The book brings these two dimensions together, linking inequalities in people's health and longevity to broader inequalities in their life chances and living standards. It does so by exploring a pervasive and persisting form of inequality. *Unequal Lives* focuses on socio-economic inequality: on inequalities across life and in death associated with inequalities in people's access to the resources needed to do well in the societies in which they live. Its primary orientation is to rich societies and to the United Kingdom (UK)[1] in particular. But the book is set in the context of broader global inequalities in people's lives.

In agrarian societies, including today's low-income countries, the critical resources for social and material success include property (land, animals and farming materials, for example). In high-income societies like the UK and the United States of America (USA), educational qualifications, rewarding occupations and high incomes are more likely to guarantee high living standards. But across these different societies, inequalities in living conditions are associated with inequalities in health. Thus, lives are at their shortest and health is at its poorest among the individuals, households and communities in the poorest circumstances. Those in somewhat better circumstances enjoy better health across longer lives – but fail to reach the levels of health achieved by those with the greatest command over their society's wealth-generating assets. In other words, there is a graded relationship between people's living conditions and their health: what is commonly referred to as a health gradient.

*Unequal Lives* investigates the enduring connection between unequal socio-economic circumstances and unequal health. It does so in order to understand why, even in societies like the UK which enjoy unparalleled levels of wealth and health, the chances of living a long and healthy life remain so unequal.

A book concerned with unravelling causes may seem out of place in a policy world where the priority is finding solutions. The emphasis today is on taking action not on deepening understanding. Explaining can be – and often is – seen as antithetical to doing, a distraction from the real business of rolling out interventions. Since 1997, rolling out interventions has been high on the UK government agenda. In other rich societies, both in Europe and beyond, governments are also investing in strategies to tackle health inequalities. But the evidence to date is not encouraging. There is little sign that socio-economic inequalities in health are narrowing. England provides an example. The raft of interventions introduced since 1997 have yet to achieve a reduction in these inequalities. Instead, trends point to a widening of inequalities in the dimensions of health on which England's health inequalities targets are based: life expectancy at birth and infant mortality. England is not alone; widening inequalities in health are also reported in other rich societies.

Part of the reason for the lack of progress may lie in the fact that too little, rather than too much, attention has been paid to understanding the social determinants of health inequalities. As a result, the current range of interventions may be literally 'off target'. They may only partially and tangentially touch the factors which underlie socio-economic inequalities in health. An intervention which fails to reach these underlying factors runs the risk of consolidating the health inequalities which it sets out to reduce. If this is the case, then a book investigating the causes of, and the connections between, unequal socio-economic circumstances and unequal health is both important and timely.

This book is an investigation undertaken for those without specialist knowledge of research on social and health inequalities. The aim is not to provide an encyclopaedia of these research fields but to draw out broad themes which link them. This approach is unlikely to impress the cognoscente. But hopefully it will provide less expert readers with an insight into how inequalities in people's health are forged through the processes which maintain socio-economic inequalities in and across their lives.

## What the book explores

An exploration of the links between people's unequal health and unequal lives takes the book into two broad research fields, one oriented to health inequalities and the other to social inequalities. It may be helpful to say a little about each.

*Research on health inequalities* is grounded in social epidemiology. As its name suggests, social epidemiology is a subfield of epidemiology, a discipline concerned with the health of populations. Epidemiology has its roots in the medical sciences: social epidemiology is the branch which links it to the social sciences. Social epidemiologists ask questions about the social patterning of population health: about its distribution across social groups. They have asked questions particularly about the health of groups who are more and less advantaged with respect to their living and working conditions. In other words, they have been concerned about the distribution of health across socio-economic groups. Social epidemiologists have trawled for evidence of links between people's socio-economic conditions and their health using historical archives and contemporary studies, including longitudinal studies which follow people over time and across their lives.

Across these data sources, the primary orientation has been to the individual. Living and working conditions – as measured by educational level, occupational status, housing conditions and income for example – have therefore tended to be seen as attributes of individuals, rather than as features of the societies of which they are part. Focusing on individuals, the search for potential causes of poor health has been restricted to factors which can be measured using information collected from them. As a result, behavioural risk factors, like cigarette smoking, tend to figure prominently in explanations of how poor circumstances are linked to high rates of diseases.

The painstaking work of social epidemiologists has highlighted the persistence of health inequalities, both over time and across changes in the major causes of death. A recurrent finding is that improving the overall health of the population does not eliminate the health disadvantages of disadvantaged groups: marked differences in the health of poorer and richer people remain despite the fact that everyone is living longer and healthier lives. Epidemiological studies have demonstrated, too, that health inequalities endure despite changes in diseases which kill. As Chapters 5 and 6 make clear, the link between wealth and health is evident both when death rates are high and infectious diseases are major killers, and when death rates are low and chronic diseases are the primary causes of death. These patterns have been revealed through studies based in the richer regions of the world. But they are being repeated on a global scale, with the burden of chronic disease increasingly borne by poorer countries and by poorer groups within them.

*Research on social inequalities* is resourced by a different cluster of disciplines, grounded in the social rather than clinical sciences. The disciplines of social policy and sociology provide the primary home for this research. Both disciplines have a long-standing concern with the social consequences of economic change in northern Europe and North America, and particularly with the impact of economic change on the lives of 'the haves and the have nots'. Like social epidemiology, the disciplines of sociology and social policy are concerned with individuals. But they are also concerned with how individual lives and individual well-being are shaped by the wider structures of society, and particularly by its labour market, education system and welfare state.

This dual orientation to individuals and to structures has made research on socio-economic inequality central to the development of the disciplines of sociology and social policy. Through the late nineteenth century, the focus was on the social consequences of the shift from an agricultural to an industrial economy. Researchers traced the effects of this shift on those who produced the country's wealth and those who owned it, noting that the costs of economic change were disproportionately borne by the wealth producers, labouring in the coal mines, steel foundries, textile mills and factories. As the twentieth century progressed, it was the loss of this industrial base – the decline of mining and shipbuilding, textile production and car manufacturing – and the emergence of 'post-industrial societies' which shaped the research agenda of sociology and social policy. Post-industrial societies have been variously defined. But they are typically characterized as ones in which manual work and large-scale industrial production no longer drive the economy, and national wealth relies instead on non-manual work in the expanding service sector (retail services, financial services and information technologies, health and welfare services, and so on). A series of studies have documented the persistence of inequality through and despite these major economic changes. The studies highlight how inequalities in people's educational attainment, employment opportunities and living standards endure, even in the richest societies where educational levels, employment rates and incomes are high and there is seemingly plenty for all. Across the last 30 years, for example, average income in the UK has risen to unprecedented levels. But over these decades inequalities in the incomes of richer and poorer households have widened sharply. It is a persisting UK trend: the gap between rich and poor has continued to widen into the new century.

The rise, and subsequent decline, of the industrial economy has left rich societies culturally richer and more diverse than they were. Across Europe, as in North America, ethnic diversity has increased. In the UK, around one in ten of the population classified themselves as non-white in the 2001 Census (APHO, 2005). High-income societies also embrace a broader range of household structures and patterns of family life than they did in the past. For example, in the early 1960s, around 5 per cent of UK births were to women who were not married; today, over 40 per cent of children are born outside marriage (Jones, 1991; ONS, 2005). But across these major social changes, children's social origins continue to shape their social destinations, a pattern found in both minority and majority ethnic groups. Thus, as later chapters discuss, children born to poorer parents enjoy less educational success and therefore do less well in the labour market than children of richer parents. The chapters point, too, to evidence that family background matters more today in the UK than it did 20 years ago in determining educational achievement and occupation. What this means is that advantage and disadvantage are increasingly transmitted across generations – and, specifically, transmitted from parents to children.

Not surprisingly, these trends have raised questions about what governments can do to reduce socio-economic inequalities. Some analyses suggest that they can do very little to narrow the gap in life chances and living standards, with the growth of the global economy further limiting their room for manoeuvre. Others point out that economies, whether national or global, are not exogenous systems which lie beyond the influence of governments. Instead, economies are fashioned and supported by policy processes. Rich countries, in particular, exercise considerable leverage over the inequalities which national and global markets produce. Their governments have policy instruments, like the tax and social security systems, which can level-up incomes between poorer and richer groups and ensure that the circumstances in which children grow up are not wholly dependent on how much parents earn or how much wealth they have inherited. But in the 1980s and 1990s, these systems became less pro-poor in countries like the UK and the USA which pursued free-market economic and social policies. It is a policy shift which has played an important role in the widening gap between rich and poor in both countries.

## Building bridges between research on health and socio-economic inequalities

This brief overview of research on social inequalities and research on health inequalities suggests that both are needed for understanding life's inequalities. We require social research to shed light on the how inequalities in people's socio-economic circumstances are produced across people's lives – and epidemiological studies to map how people's socio-economic circumstances affect their health. While important gaps remain, there is an extensive body of evidence addressing these questions.

But across the last 150 years, the two research fields have largely remained separate. Research on the causes of socio-economic inequality (typically called class inequality) has continued to be concentrated in the disciplines of sociology and social policy. Meanwhile, research on the causes of socio-economic inequalities in health is being driven forward by social epidemiologists. Relatively little work has been done across the boundaries of these two research fields. More work across these boundaries is needed for a number of reasons.

First, as the chapters of the book make clear, embedding research on socio-economic inequalities in health within research on socio-economic inequalities deepens our understanding of the persistence of health inequalities. It is very hard to explain health inequalities without this broader societal perspective: very hard to understand how health inequalities persist over time and across generations without an understanding of how socio-economic inequalities are maintained over time and across generations.

This deeper understanding is required not only for its own sake. Building bridges between social and health research is important, second, to inform judgements about whether health inequalities are unjust and unfair. As Chapter 1 notes, philosophers suggest that inequalities in health are unfair and unjust if they stem from inequalities in the opportunities and resources to which every individual should have access. It is an argument which is grounded in ethical principle but can only be tested through empirical research. The ethical principle is that everyone matters equally. Systemic inequalities in people's life chances and health chances, therefore, violate this principle of moral equality. Empirical research is needed to investigate whether there are systemic inequalities in people's life chances, and whether these systemic inequalities give rise to inequalities in their chances of good health. The book interrogates the evidence.

Bridge-building is required, third, for the development of policies capable of tackling socio-economic inequalities in health. There is widespread agreement that these inequalities can not be addressed through health policies alone. Other policies – education and employment policies, fiscal and welfare policies – play the decisive role in equalizing the opportunities and resources which determine people's health. This suggests that health and social policies need to operate in concert if they are to make a positive impact on health inequalities. But intersectoral solutions to health inequalities are hard to deliver without interdisciplinary understandings of their causes. In other words, joined-up policies require joined-up science. A World Health Organization report reinforces this point. To tackle socio-economic inequalities in health 'new forms of equity-focused multidisciplinary research are needed to support a multisectoral policy approach' (WHO 2004: 9).

Studies which follow people over time and across their lives, provide a key resource for building equity-oriented multidisciplinary perspectives. These longitudinal studies enable researchers to track how people's social circumstances and health chances are shaped across the course of their lives. Such studies are informing what is called a 'life course perspective' which locates people in their social and health biographies. It is through this life course perspective that understandings of social and health inequalities are starting to converge. For example, both sociologists and epidemiologists are highlighting how the conditions in which children are brought up have lifelong effects on their socio-economic position and health, effects which in turn determine the conditions in which the future generation of children are born. Life course perspectives therefore provide a cornerstone of the book.

## Challenges to bridge-building

Building bridges between research on social and health inequalities is a project with some major challenges.

One challenge is that disciplines have their own vocabularies. Concepts with similar meanings are differently described. Thus, social epidemiologists tend to refer to socio-economic position and socio-economic groups, while sociologists have traditionally preferred to talk of social class and social classes. Epidemiologists often refer to people's diets and patterns of physical activity, together with habits like cigarette smoking, as 'health behaviours' and 'risk factors'. Because these behaviours and factors can be directly linked to people's health, they are characterized as 'proximal causes' (in proximity to the outcome). Terms like 'risk factors' and 'proximal causes' are rarely found in sociological accounts. While health behaviour is still used, sociological studies are increasingly turning to terms like 'social practices' and 'identity practices', which signal how patterns of diet, exercise and smoking are embedded in people's social relations and their sense of self. Differences in vocabulary, of course, signal deeper differences in perspective. Aware that readers may feel themselves sinking in these shifting disciplinary sands, the book offers broad overviews of key perspectives and (hopefully!) simple definitions of key terms.

A second challenge is that large sections of these fields lie uncharted. Most of what is known about social and health inequalities derives from data on individuals, and not from studies of the social institutions which shape their lives. People are continually stratified as they make their way through the education system, the labour market and the welfare state – yet these stratifying processes are hard to capture in surveys of individuals. Further, the individuals invited to take part in surveys are disproportionately drawn from rich societies, which are home to only one in six of the world's population. Research within these societies is biased towards white men. Thus, research in the UK has only begun to track how socio-economic inequalities are manifested in women's lives and women's health – and how socio-economic and gender inequalities are mediated by ethnicity. In all societies, information relating to sexuality is even sparser. With so little information on these core dimensions of inequality, research can tell us little about how, singly and together, they shape people's health.

A third challenge is that, while there are many empty spaces on the research canvas, it is nonetheless vast. Selecting themes and simplifying findings has been an essential part of writing the book, with references provided for readers looking to open doors to the larger pool of research on which the book draws. The need to restrict coverage means that there are important areas which are not covered in detail. The book focuses on socio-economic inequality but does not deal in depth with its intersections with other dimensions of inequality: for example, with the different ways in which socio-economic inequality works its way into the lives of men and women and how these processes are additionally influenced by ethnic identity and sexuality.

It needs to be noted, too, that research on social and health inequalities is dominated by quantitative studies in which those in the most advantaged circumstances are taken as the reference group against which other groups are compared. The strength of this approach is that it succinctly captures the scale of health inequalities. It tells us, for example, that children in the UK growing up in the poorest conditions are twice as likely to die in the first year of life (see Chapter 2). It also puts the emphasis on levelling up: on lifting standards of health in poorer groups closer to those in the most advantaged group. But there are drawbacks to measuring inequalities by comparing patterns in poorer groups against those in the best-off group. For those without a strong statistical background, much higher risks can appear to imply that the adverse outcome is very likely to happen. As discussed in later chapters, an elevated risk for poorer children reveals only that they are more vulnerable than children in richer families, not that they are certain to succumb: in rich societies, many adverse outcomes, like death in the first year of life, are rare even in the poorest groups. Further, taking the most privileged group as the reference category can mean that their lives and lifestyles are not put under the spotlight. The gaze of researchers and policy-makers can shift away from advantages enjoyed by the well-off and focus instead on what, by comparison, appear to be the deficiencies of poorer groups.

These challenges mean that the book is far from the final word on the connections between social and health inequalities. Its aims are much more modest. It hopes to provide a range of tools for understanding the links between socio-economic inequalities in people's lives and in their health in rich societies like the UK. The chapters which follow seek to provide these tools by introducing some useful *concepts*, summarizing some illuminating *evidence* and forging some deeper *understandings* of the links between inequalities in people's lives and inequalities in people's health. The importance of policy runs as a recurrent theme through these analyses, and is explicitly addressed in Chapter 11.

## What the chapters are about

The book explores socio-economic inequalities in the lives people lead and the health that they enjoy. It does so through chapters which provide linked but freestanding analyses: conceptual, empirical and explanatory. While the chapters form a series of stepping stones, each leading on to the next, they can also be read separately. It is therefore hoped that the reader can 'pick and mix' their way through the book.

*Part 1 (Chapters 1 to 4)* introduce the *concepts* which mark out the intellectual territory of the book. Chapter 1 looks at the concepts of health inequalities and health equity, the later discussion taking in philosophical insights into what makes health inequalities unfair and unjust. Chapter 2 provides a short review of measures of health and health inequalities. Among the indicators it discusses are those based on mortality, self-assessed health and limiting long-term illness, as well as on measures of the development of health in childhood and its decline through middle age.

Chapters 3 and 4 turn to the concepts of socio-economic inequality and socio-economic position, and to measures of socio-economic position. Chapter 3 explores what can be learned from sociological research on socio-economic inequality. The rich seam of studies suggests that inequalities in socio-economic position are both imposed by the social structure and produced by people as they live their lives. Chapter 4 discusses the problems and pitfalls of measuring socio-economic position, and introduces some of its most widely used indicators. These include measures based on individual and household characteristics, like education, occupation and income, and measures based on information about the places in which people live.

*Part 2 (Chapters 5 and 6)* is concerned with *patterns* of socio-economic inequalities in health. Chapter 5 considers evidence of inequalities across countries and over time, discussing both global inequalities and historical trends in Britain. Chapter 6 turns to examine health inequalities within countries and across changes in patterns of disease. In early industrializing societies like the UK and the USA, changes in patterns of diet and tobacco consumption have been largely endogenous, driven by developments in their own domestic economies. However, the increasing international dominance of high-income societies has resulted in the export of the economic systems and patterns of consumption on which their wealth is founded. It is a globalizing process which has triggered rapid changes in the lives and lifestyles of the much larger populations of low- and middle-income countries.

*Part 3 (Chapters 7 to 11)* focuses on building *understandings* of socio-economic and health inequalities. Chapter 7 discusses the concept of the social determinants of health, a concept central both to health research and health policy. It notes that researchers have identified social position, and socio-economic position in particular, as a fundamental determinant of health. Chapters 8 and 9 focus on this fundamental determinant, investigating how inequalities in people's socio-economic position are reproduced over their lives and across generations. The chapters look in turn at the influence of family background on educational attainment and occupation (Chapter 8) and on partnership and parenthood (Chapter 9). Chapter 10 draws on research which maps how people's social conditions, from before birth and across childhood and adulthood, influence how their health develops through childhood – and declines in later life.

Across the chapters of the book, evidence is noted of how policies, both national and global, can work to reduce or to widen inequalities in people's life chances and living standards. Chapter 11 focuses on the welfare systems of high-income countries to gain greater insight into their redistributive effects.

It presents evidence on how these policies can combine to distribute income from richer to poorer groups.

The book ends with a short conclusion which returns to the ethical challenge of promoting equal lives, and the policy mechanisms through which governments can make progress towards this goal.

# PART 1
## Key Terms

Part 1 provides an overview of the concepts and measures which underpin research on people's unequal lives. Chapter 1 focuses on the concepts of health inequalities and health equity, while Chapter 2 discusses key measures of health and health inequalities. Chapters 3 and 4 turn to the concept and measurement of socio-economic position. Across these chapters, particular attention is paid to measures used in the UK.

# 1 Health inequalities and inequities

## 1.1 Introduction

What is meant by health inequalities varies between countries and changes over time. In some countries, the term is rarely used. In the USA, it has not been widely taken up by either researchers or policy-makers, with the term 'health disparities' preferred instead. In the UK, the concept of health inequalities fell out of favour with government in the 1980s and early 1990s but currently occupies a pivotal place in the policy discourse. In New Zealand, ethnic inequalities are described as health inequalities, while in Britain, as in Europe more generally, health inequalities are more likely to refer to inequalities in the health of socio-economic groups. Section 1.2 provides a guide to this maze of meanings. It suggests that three broad understandings of health inequalities can be identified. The concept can be used to draw attention to health differences between individuals, health differences between population groups and health differences between those occupying unequal positions in the dominant social hierarchies.

The second part of the chapter turns to the concept of health inequity. Widely regarded as a normative concept, 'health inequity' is a term applied to health inequalities which are judged to be unfair and unjust. Understanding what is unfair and unjust about health inequities takes us beyond health research into moral and political philosophy, where a long-running debate about equality and justice has generated a large and complex literature. Section 1.3 takes a selective approach to this literature. It discusses insights from perspectives whose influence has rippled out from philosophy and into health research and social policy. Some readers may choose to skip this section, moving straight onto Chapter 2. For others, an appreciation of ethical debates will be integral to their broader understanding of social and health inequalities.

## 1.2 What are health inequalities?

The terms 'health inequality' and 'health inequalities' tend to be used inter-changeably in national and international policy debates. Thus, for example, England's 1999 White Paper on public health used the singular form, speaking of 'health inequality (which) runs throughout life, from birth through to old age' (Secretary of State for Health, 1999: 41). The follow-up White Paper, published in 2004, pluralized the concept and referred to 'inequalities in health . . . (with) health and life expectancy not shared equally across the population' (Secretary of State for Health, 2004: 10). The plural usage is more common. The book follows this convention. The pluralized form ('health inequalities') is used to signal that both social inequalities, and the dimensions of health with which they are associated, are multiple.

There is a voluminous and ever-expanding literature on the concept of health inequalities, its size indicative of the lack of agreement about what the term means. For those not immersed in the definitional debates, it can be all too easy to lose one's way. Box 1.1 therefore provides a simplified guide. It suggests that understandings of health inequalities take three broad forms.

Health inequalities can be cast as individual differences in health, differences in health between population groups and differences between groups linked to broader social inequalities. These definitions are distinguished by their focus on individuals (individual differences in health), the social groups to which individuals belong (health differences between population groups) and the unequal structures of which groups are part (health differences between unequal groups). The three concepts are used to describe within country inequalities: to capture health inequalities between individuals and groups living in the same country. They can also be applied to inequalities in health at the global level.

---

**Box 1.1**

Three meanings of health inequalities:

- health differences between individuals
- health differences between population groups
- health differences between groups occupying unequal positions in society

---

### Health differences between individuals

For some policy analysts, health inequalities simply refer to differences in the health of individuals. It is a shorthand way of saying that some individuals are ill and some are not, some live long lives and others do not. As this suggests, the focus is on the individual: he or she is the unit of analysis. It is therefore the distribution of health between individuals, and not the distribution of health across social groups, which is being described. Thus health inequalities are 'the variations in health status across individuals in a population' with individuals ranged along a continuum from 'best health to worst health' (Murray *et al.*, 1999: 537). Box 1.2 gives other examples of this way of defining health inequalities.

Figure 1.1 provides an illustration of what the distribution of health across individuals looks like. It describes the variation in health status in England based on people's self-assessment of their health (as very good, good, fair, bad or very bad). It suggests that the distribution is heavily skewed towards the 'good health' end of the continuum, with a relatively small proportion of the population in the 'less than good' categories (Sproston and Primatesta 2004).

The individual differences in health which Figure 1.1 reveals have been called 'pure health inequalities' because they relate to only one dimension

---

**Box 1.2**

'Health inequality should be defined in terms of inequality across individuals. By moving towards the measurement of the distribution of health across individuals, the study of inequality will be put on a firmer scientific footing.' (Murray *et al.*, 1999: 541)

'The approach defines health inequality as the uneven distribution of health across all units in a population, independent of population subgroup.' (Goesling and Firebaugh, 2004: 132)

---

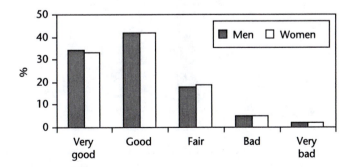

**Figure 1.1**   Self-assessed health, adults aged 16 and over, England 2003
*Source:* adapted from Sproston and Primatesta, 2004, table 10.1

(health), rather than two (health and social group) (Wagstaff and van Doorlaer 2000). Those favouring this approach have therefore needed to find a different term for differences between groups. 'Social group health differences' have been proposed (Murray *et al.*, 1999: 537).

A pure health inequalities approach was advocated within the World Health Organization (WHO) for a brief period in the late 1990s and early 2000s. It also featured in the WHO's *2000 World Health Report* (WHO 2000). The focus on the individual, rather than the social, patterning of health, was widely criticized (see for example, Braveman *et al.*, 2000, 2001; Evans *et al.*, 2001). By appropriating a concept widely understood to refer to inequalities in the health of less and more advantaged groups, the approach was seen to confuse rather than clarify the policy agenda. Specifically, it was seen to deflect national and international attention away from the unequal distribution of health and the broader social inequalities which underlie it. Tellingly perhaps, the WHO quickly abandoned this concept of health inequalities (Braveman, 2006).

## Health differences between population groups

The second approach draws attention to the social patterning of health. It moves beyond an emphasis on variations in the health of individuals to acknowledge health differences between groups. These groups can be defined by a range of criteria, including age, gender and socio-economic position. As one example, Figure 1.2 maps the distribution of health by household income, charting the proportion of adults in different income quintiles who rate their health as 'not good' (that is, as fair, bad or very bad). As it

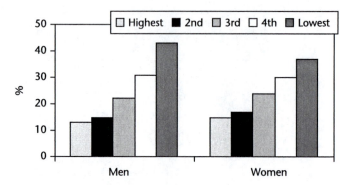

**Figure 1.2** Proportion of women and men aged 16 and over assessing their health as 'not good' (as fair, bad or very bad) by income quintile based on equivalized household income, England 2003

*Source:* adapted from Sproston and Primatesta, 2004, table 10.3

indicates, the proportion climbs from around 15 per cent in the richest fifth of households to around 40 per cent in the poorest households (Sproston and Primatesta, 2004).

Box 1.3 includes extracts from major policy documents in the UK and US, together with a report produced by the primary US health research funding agency, to illustrate the distinctive features of this second approach. As the examples suggest, health differences linked to people's socio-economic position, gender and ethnicity are acknowledged. These differences are recognized to 'occur', with variations in health status 'associated with a range of factors'. But a connection between these health differences and social inequalities is not made explicit.

As Box 1.3 indicates, the language underplays any potential link between differences in people's health and inequalities in their social position. In the three extracts, the emphasis is therefore on 'variations' and 'disparities' in the health of 'different groups' and 'population segments'. This careful phrasing has been adopted in contexts where researchers and governments are reluctant to speak openly about social inequalities. Under the New Right government in power in Britain in the 1980s and 1990s, for example, 'inequalities' was a proscribed term. Policy documents were, however, able to acknowledge 'variations'. Framed in this way, it was possible for the government to acknowledge 'the particular needs and concerns of specific groups of people in the population' including 'the different needs of people in different socioeconomic groups' (Secretary of State for Health, 1992: 116 and 122). In the USA, the concept of health disparities can be seen as serving a similar function,

---

**Box 1.3**

'There are variations in health in the extent of sickness and premature death between different groups within the population. Some groups can expect to enjoy substantially better health and longer lives than others. These variations in health status are associated with a range of often interacting factors: geography, socio-economic status, gender, environment, ethnicity, culture, and lifestyle.' (Variations SubGroup, 1995: 5)

'Health disparities [exist] among segments of the population, including differences which occur by gender, race or ethnicity, education or income, disability, geographic location, or sexual orientation.' (DHHS, 2000: 7)

'Racial and ethnic minorities, poor people, and other groups experience worse health in a variety of circumstances. Called health disparities, these differences are reflected by indices such as excess mortality and morbidity and shorter life expectancy.' (Thomson *et al.*, 2006: 15)

appealing to a scientific and policy constituency who may be uncomfortable with the concept and reality of social inequalities. As one major research review put it, 'the term "health disparities" is widely used to describe differences in health status without necessarily implying the presence of injustice' (Thomson *et al.*, 2006: 25). Perhaps for this reason, the concept of health disparities has quickly gained widespread currency in the USA (Adler, 2006), figuring centrally in the country's public health strategy, *Healthy People 2010* (DHHS, 2000).

### Health differences between groups occupying unequal positions in society

A third approach turns the spotlight on the connection between people's health and their position in the social hierarchies around which societies are built. In other words, health inequalities are health differences associated with social inequalities. Examples of this approach are given in Box 1.4.

While the term 'health inequalities' is widely used both within the UK and internationally, it has yet to be incorporated into the vocabulary of US research and policy. Instead, the research and policy community has stayed with 'health disparities'. Those wishing to signal the link between health disparities and social inequalities do so by making clear that health disparities refer to health differences 'between social groups who have different levels of underlying social advantage/disadvantage – that is, different positions in a social hierarchy' (Braveman and Gruskin, 2003: 254).

In some countries, like New Zealand, the term 'health inequalities' has become incorporated into the policy vocabulary to highlight, and to mobilize action around, ethnic differences in health and, in particular, differences between the indigenous Maori community and the colonizing white com-

---

**Box 1.4**

'Social inequalities (or inequities) in health refer to health disparities, within and between countries ... that systematically burden populations rendered vulnerable by underlying social structures and political, economic, and legal institutions.' (Krieger, 2001: 698)

'Health disparities/inequalities do not refer to all differences in health. A health disparity/inequality is a particular type of difference in health ... it is a difference in which disadvantaged social groups – such as the poor, racial/ethnic minorities, women, or other groups who have persistently experienced social disadvantage or discrimination – systematically experience worse health or greater health risks than more advantaged social groups.' (Braveman, 2006: 167)

munity (Humpage and Fleras, 2001). However, in most countries, health inequalities are defined in terms of socio-economic inequalities in health, whether measured at the individual level (by a person's education or occupation, for example) or the area level (for instance, by the level of deprivation in the neighbourhood in which they live). In the UK, health inequalities which relate to other structures of inequality – like gender or ethnicity – are typically labelled in these terms: as gender inequalities in health, ethnic inequalities in health, and so on. In cross-national analyses too, 'health inequalities' typically refer to the systematic differences in health captured by measures of education, occupation and income. An example of this general pattern is given in Box 1.5.

The three meanings of health inequalities – as individual variations, group differences and socially structured inequalities – are not mutually exclusive. In all societies, the health of different individuals is different, health varies between social groups and many of these group differences reflect deep-rooted inequalities in people's lives. All three dimensions could therefore be studied at the same time. However, researchers and policy analysts tend to favour one of these approaches. For example, those interested in individual variations tend to be less concerned about group differences, while those concerned about group differences may well resist linking them to socially structured inequalities.

The book follows this pattern, focusing on one of the three concepts of health inequalities. It uses the term to refer not to individual health differences or to group health disparities, but to the health consequences of systemic inequalities. As the book's subtitle signals, it focuses on the connections between socio-economic inequalities in people's lives and their health. It is a focus which raises questions about the nature of these inequalities and why they persist even in rich societies enjoying high standards of health. These questions are explored in the chapters which follow. But running through the book's discussion of the 'what' and 'why' of health inequalities are deeper ethical questions about the injustice of these inequalities. It is to some of these questions that the chapter now briefly turns.

---

**Box 1.5**

'At the start of the 21st century, all European countries are faced with substantial inequalities in the health of their populations. People with a lower level of education, a lower occupational class, or a lower level of income tend to die at a younger age, and to have a higher prevalence of most types of health problem.' (Mackenbach, 2005a: 3)

## 1.3 What are health inequities?

For most health researchers and policy analysts, the concept of health inequalities is a descriptive one. Whether applied to individual differences, social variations or socially structured inequalities, the term 'health inequalities' is used to describe patterns of health. Simply describing what is, it makes no moral judgements about what should be (Evans *et al.*, 2001). In contrast, health inequity is widely regarded as a normative concept. It refers to health inequalities which are 'politically, socially and economically unacceptable' (WHO, 1978: 1). As Margaret Whitehead notes, 'the term inequity has a moral and ethical dimension' (1990: 5). It is applied to health differences which 'are unfair and unjust' (Whitehead, 1990: 5).

Individual health differences are not usually couched in these terms. Most people accept as inevitable that health will vary between one individual and another, and between the same individual at different points in their life. Differences between undifferentiated individuals are therefore unlikely to be seen as unfair and unjust. Similarly, group disparities in health which are unrelated to broader social divisions tend not to be cast as health inequities. Poorer health among older than younger adults, for example, is more likely to be seen as a biological inevitability than as a social injustice. It is socially structured inequalities in health which are most commonly judged as inequitable.

It is worth pausing and reflecting on why health differences associated with broader social inequalities qualify as health inequities. Answers which tell us that socio-economic inequalities are inequitable because they are unfair and unjust, do not help very much. This is because equity, justice and fairness are commonly treated as synonyms, with each defined in terms of the others (Le Grand, 1991). Thus, the concept of fairness is invoked to explain what is equitable – and equity is understood as that which is fair and just. Trying to move beyond this circularity of terms takes us beyond the disciplines of sociology and social epidemiology which are driving forward understandings of social and health inequalities. It takes us into philosophy and ethics, disciplines centrally engaged in debating what is meant by equity and justice.

These debates have been going on for centuries. They have yet to reach a conclusion. Their complexity means that discussions of equity and justice are hard to follow by those not trained in philosophy. But the debates are yielding insights which are too important to be left outside the boundaries of health research. The next two subsections consider some of these insights. One theme concerns what is called moral equality and the basic freedoms which are needed to ensure everyone is accorded the same consideration and respect. A second, and closely related, theme concerns the role of social structures and institutions in determining whether everyone shares equally in these basic freedoms.

It needs to be emphasized that the subsections do not provide an overview of the work on which they draw. Thus they note the influence of John Rawls, but do not outline his theory of justice or the set of foundational principles on which it is based. Readers seeking a summary of this work should look elsewhere (for example, Freeman, 2002). The subsections have a more specific purpose: to trawl contemporary philosophy for recurrent themes which have particular relevance for health. For, while philosophers and political theorists clearly disagree about many issues, these disagreements appear to have their origins in deeper points of agreement.

## Moral equality and basic freedoms

First, philosophers agree that everyone is morally equal. Philosophers have long since moved away from the idea that there is a natural human hierarchy, in which one individual or one group is inherently superior to another. Instead, political and moral philosophy is built on what Will Kymlicka calls an 'egalitarian plateau' (2002: 4). The starting point is that each person has the same moral worth and therefore everyone's life and life prospects matter equally. This moral equality means that I matter as much as you, and we both deserve as much consideration and respect as everyone else. In making people's equal moral worth a cornerstone of their theories, philosophers are seen to be reflecting as well as informing public opinion (Kymlicka, 2002). Thus, it is not only philosophical treatises which have long been grounded in the principle of moral equality: so, too, have constitutional and legal systems. In the eighteenth century, it underpinned the US *Declaration of Independence* and France's *Declaration of the Rights of Man*. Today, it frames the *Universal Declaration on Human Rights* and the *European Convention on Human Rights and Fundamental Freedoms*.

Second, philosophers agree that the principle of moral equality requires that we all enjoy the same basic freedoms. Without what the European Convention calls fundamental freedoms, moral equality remains an aspiration; with these freedoms, it has a chance of becoming a reality. Societies which endorse the principle of moral equality should therefore be ones which strive to equalize people's basic freedoms 'since citizens of a just society are to have the same basic rights' (Rawls, 1999: 61). Such societies would see inequalities in basic freedoms as violating the principle of moral equality. They would therefore be seen as inequitable (unfair and unjust).

While most philosophers agree that justice requires that people are accorded equal basic freedoms, they disagree about the form that these basic freedoms should take. What needs to be equally distributed to make a society just? This is the 'equality of what?' question (Sen, 1980). It is here that philosophical debate begins in earnest and the disagreements start to emerge. This is because, as Sen notes, 'the real work begins with the specification of what it is that is to be equalised' (Sen, 2004b: 22). This real work has produced two broad answers to the question 'equality of what?' One emphasizes the importance of equality in what people have; the other argues for equality in what they can be and achieve. These different standpoints are associated respectively with the work of John Rawls, a philosopher, and Amartya Sen, a polymath whose expertise ranges across philosophy, economics and history.

Rawls introduces the concept of 'primary social goods' to mark out the basic freedoms which would be equalized in his vision of a just society. The concept is a broad and imprecise one: 'the primary social goods, to give them in broad categories, are rights and liberties, opportunities and powers, income and wealth' (Rawls, 1999: 92). They are primary goods because they constitute the minimum set of rights and resources that individuals need to be able to participate as equals in the society of which they are a part. They are social goods because the existence and distribution of these rights and resources is determined by the major institutions of society. As Rawls puts it, 'they are social goods in view of their connection with the basic structure' (1999: 92).

Sen takes issue with Rawls's conceptualization of equal basic freedoms as a set of primary goods. This, he suggests, is too narrow a view. He points out that people can be accorded the same primary goods – for example, they can all have the right to vote and all be given the same income – but remain deeply unequal. Differences between people and in their circumstances mean that they will require different quantities and combinations of primary goods to secure basic freedoms that are of equal value to them. Sen gives the example of two people, one with and one without impairments, who will not enjoy equal freedom simply by being given the same basket of primary goods. Differently weighted baskets are likely to be required to achieve equality in basic freedoms (see Sen, 1980, 1999). For instance, the individual with impairments may require greater educational opportunities and a higher income to secure the same life chances as one without impairments. As another example, Chapter 8 discusses how children from privileged backgrounds – with parents who have professional jobs and high incomes – derive more benefit from their right to education than children from poorer families: they convert their years of compulsory schooling into more educational qualifications and thus higher status jobs and higher incomes.

With such examples in mind, Sen concludes that the focus of ethical debate needs to move away from primary goods to 'what the person is doing and achieving' (1984: 84). In other words, equality in people's formal rights and freedoms is not enough; they need to be backed up with equality in what he calls substantive freedoms or capabilities. He therefore argues that what matters is not 'primary goods (as demanded by Rawls) but . . . the substantive freedoms – the capabilities – to choose a life one has reason to value' (Sen, 1999: 74). This central message is conveyed in Box 1.6. In Sen's vision of a

---

**Box 1.6**

---

'What a person is free to have, not just what he or she actually has, is relevant, I have argued, to a theory of justice.' (Sen, 2004a: 335)

'Primary goods themselves are mainly various types of general resources . . . An alternative . . . is to concentrate on the *actual living* that people manage to achieve (or going beyond that, on the *freedom* to achieve actual livings one has reason to value).' (Sen, 1999: 73, emphasis in original)

---

just society, governments would seek to achieve equality in people's freedoms to be, do and achieve.

As these brief summaries suggest, Rawls and Sen provide different perspectives on what needs to be equally distributed to make a society just. What light do these perspectives shed on health and health inequities?

At first glance, Rawls's work has little to say either about health or about health inequities. He expressly excludes health and what he calls 'vigour' as primary goods because, 'although their possession is influenced by the basic structure, they are not directly under its control' (Rawls, 1999: 62). Seeing health more as a matter of luck, he designs his principles of justice on the assumption that everyone is in good health and no one dies prematurely. It has been left to other theorists to explore what his ethical schema would mean if it were applied to real-world societies in which good health is not equally shared by all. Norman Daniels has made a particularly important contribution here. He argues that the philosophical concept of primary social goods is analogous to the epidemiological concept of the social determinants of health: Rawls's 'broad categories' of primary goods – like opportunities, income and wealth – describe broad sets of social factors known to have a determining influence on people's health (Daniels *et al.*, 1999). As Daniels puts it, there is 'a correspondence between the key determinants of health and the primary social goods included in his index and governed by his principles' (2002: 263). Daniels therefore concludes that the primary goods to be equally distributed in a just society would include those which determine health.[1] In other words, 'access to health resources is a basic freedom and therefore health access should be distributed equally in the ideal society' (Bommier and Stecklov, 2002: 503). This extension of Rawls's perspective suggests that inequalities in people's access to health resources violate the fundamental principle of equal basic freedoms, and are therefore inequitable (unjust and unfair).

Health figures much more centrally in Sen's capability perspective and his wider vision of social justice (Box 1.7). On the one hand, the freedom to be healthy determines other capabilities: as Sen puts it, 'we can do very little

---

**Box 1.7**

---

'Health is among the most important conditions of human life and a critically significant constituent of human capabilities which we have reason to value. Any conception of social justice that accepts the need for a fair distribution . . . of human capabilities cannot ignore the role of health in human life and the opportunities that people respectively have to achieve good health – free from escapable illness, avoidable afflictions and premature mortality. Equity in the achievement and distribution of health gets, thus, incorporated and embedded in a larger understanding of justice.' (Sen, 2004b: 23)

---

indeed if we are not alive' (Sen, 1999: 24). On the other hand, the freedom to be healthy depends on other capabilities: on the freedom to be well nourished, to be educated, to secure an income, and so on. In other words, 'different kinds of freedom inter-relate with one another, and freedom of one type may help greatly in advancing freedom of another type' (Sen, 1999: 82).

While Sen puts particular emphasis on equalizing people's opportunities to achieve good health (see Box 1.7), he has consistently argued against putting it (or any other substantive freedom) on 'a list of capabilities for all societies for all times to come' (Sen, 2004c: 78). He has resisted such a list because he sees capabilities as contingent on context. Thus, 'we may have to give priority to the ability to be well nourished when people are dying of hunger, whereas the freedom to be sheltered may rightly receive more weight when people are in general well fed, but lack shelter' (Sen, 2004c: 78). However others have argued that, while lists cannot be set in tablets of stone, it is both possible and important to specify core capabilities which a just society would seek to secure for everyone. This argument has been powerfully articulated by Martha Nussbaum. She observes that 'we need to have an account, for political purposes, of what central human capabilities are, even if we know that this account will always be contested and remade' (Nussbaum, 2003: 56). Her list of ten central capabilities is headed by 'life' and 'bodily health' (Box 1.8). It is a list which suggests that inequalities in people's chances of longevity and good health are particularly profound inequities.

Rawls and Sen are often seen to offer alternative, and competing, perspectives on equality. One seeks to equalize people's holdings of goods, the other to equalize what people are able to be and do. However, when these perspectives are applied to health, the differences begin to blur. Access to health has been identified among people's basic and fundamental freedoms by theorists working within both a goods-oriented and a capability-oriented framework. In their different ways, both approaches lend support to the principle of equal access to the resources and opportunities needed to enjoy good health

---

**Box 1.8**

---

'The Central Human Capabilities[a]

1. Life. Being able to live to the end of a human life of normal length; not dying prematurely, or before one's life is so reduced as to be not worth living.
2. Bodily Health. Being able to have good health, including reproductive health; to be adequately nourished; to have adequate shelter.' (Nussbaum, 2003: 41)

[a] First two of ten central capabilities.

---

across a life not foreshortened by premature death. Both, too, highlight the importance of the social structure in regulating access to these determinants of health.

### The importance of social structures

The traditional focus of philosophy has been on the individual. But the principle of people's moral equality which guides contemporary theory is stimulating an increasing focus on social structures. The work of Rawls and Sen has again been particularly influential. Both emphasize that a society's structure determines who enjoys, and who is denied, the freedoms which underwrite their moral equality. Both therefore put the social structure, and the social institutions through which it exerts its influence on individuals, at the centre of their analysis.

Rawls's critique of unequal social structures is framed in general terms; it is also one couched in the gendered vocabulary of 'men'. Elements of this critique are summarized in Box 1.9. In this account, he argues that 'the primary subject of justice is the basic structure of society because its effects are so profound and present from the start'. He suggests that this basic structure consists of 'various social positions' embedded in 'major social institutions'. He argues that the major institutions – and he includes the labour market and systems regulating the inheritance of property among his examples – affect people's life chances. These institutions 'influence their life-prospects, what they can expect to be and how well they can hope to do' (Rawls, 1999: 7). Social institutions have this pervasive and lifelong influence because they 'favour certain starting places over others'. As the quotation in Box 1.9 makes clear, Rawls is particularly concerned about inequalities that result from social structures which systematically advantage those occupying privileged positions within it. 'These are especially deep inequalities' (Rawls, 1999: 7).

Sen provides a more detailed account of the role of social structures in

---

**Box 1.9**

'The basic structure of society is the primary subject of justice because its effects are so profound and present from the start. The intuitive notion here is that this structure contains various social positions and that men born into different positions have different expectations of life determined, in part, by the political system as well as by economic and social circumstances. In this way, the institutions of society favor certain starting places over others. These are especially deep inequalities. Not only are they pervasive, but they affect men's initial chances in life; yet they cannot possibly be justified by an appeal to the notions of merit or desert. It is these inequalities, presumably inevitable in the basic structure of any society, to which the principles of social justice must in the first instance apply.'
(Rawls, 1999: 7)

---

influencing what Rawls calls people's starting places and chances in life. Sen has undertaken analyses of economic and social policy in richer and poorer countries, documenting how different policy regimes affect the level and distribution of basic capabilities (Drèze and Sen, 1989; Sen, 1999). Sen has drawn a contrast between two approaches. In one, economic growth is the overriding priority; in the other, enhancing capabilities is the primary goal. In the first, and more common, approach governments spend little on public services like education, health care, housing and sanitation until their countries are wealthy. The second scales up investment in these public services to build and equalize capabilities. It 'does not wait for dramatic increases in per capita levels of real income, and works through priority being given to providing social services (particularly health care and basic education) that reduce mortality and enhance quality of life' (Sen, 1999: 46). It is an approach which can combine low levels of national wealth with high levels of life expectancy (see Chapters 5 and 6). As Drèze and Sen conclude from their comparative policy analysis, 'when it comes to enhancing basic human capabilities, and in particular, beating persistent hunger and deprivation, the role played by public support – including the public delivery of health care and basic education – is hard to replace' (1989: 258).

Sen's capability approach has transformed international debates about social justice and economic policy. His work has informed and legitimated a focus on human development, rather than economic development, as the goal of national and global policies. Lead international agencies, like the United Nations, now 'speak the language' of capabilities and substantive freedoms. As Box 1.10 indicates, they are increasingly arguing for societies to be judged, not simply by how rich they are, but by how much they enhance and equalize people's capabilities.

---

**Box 1.10**

---

'Extreme inequalities in opportunities and life chances have a direct bearing on what people can be and what they can do – that is, on human capabilities . . . Rights and freedoms cannot stand alone. People are likely to be restricted in what they can do with their freedom and their rights if they are poor, ill, denied an education or lack the capacity to influence what happens to them. To be meaningful, formal equalities have to be backed up by what Amartya Sen has called "substantive freedoms" – the capabilities – to choose a way of life and do the things that one values. Deep inequalities limit these substantive freedoms, rendering hollow the idea of equality before the law.' (UNDP, 2005: 51 and 54)

---

## 1.4 Conclusions

The chapter has focused on the concepts of health inequalities and inequities. It noted that 'health inequalities' is a concept with a variety of meanings. Three influential understandings were identified: individual differences in health, social variations in health and inequalities in health linked to broader social inequalities. While not universally adopted, it is the third meaning of health inequalities which has the widest currency within the research and policy communities both within the UK and internationally. It has been applied particularly to socio-economic inequalities in health, to both inequalities between richer and poorer countries and between richer and poorer groups within countries. This is the concept of health inequalities which frames the book.

Health inequalities which are systematically related to people's unequal positions in society are often defined as health inequities, a designation given to inequalities which are considered to be unjust and unfair. While philosophy provides few simple answers, it has shed an important light on what is inequitable about these inequalities.

Guiding contemporary philosophy is the principle of moral equality, a principle which asserts that we all have equal worth and should therefore be accorded equal basic rights. The basic freedoms have been defined in different ways. Two influential approaches are represented by John Rawls and Amartya Sen. The former argues that fairness and justice require that resources and opportunities are distributed equally ('primary social goods'); the latter that they are distributed in ways which enable people to live lives which have equal value to them ('capabilities'). Taken together, these perspectives suggest that just and fair societies are those whose structures and institutions promote equality in these basic freedoms, with Sen looking beyond equality in what people have, to equality in what they can do and achieve. Unjust and unfair societies are those whose structures and institutions advance the freedoms of some to have, do and achieve at the cost of the freedoms of others.

The concepts of primary goods and capabilities can be, and have been, stretched to include access to the resources and opportunities needed for good health. This applied work suggests that health inequalities are health inequities when they stem, either directly or indirectly, from inequalities in people's basic freedoms. Judgements about whether or not this is the case cannot be made in abstract, on the basis of philosophical argument alone (Anand and Peter, 2004; Browne and Stears, 2005). Empirical evidence is also needed. Research is needed to investigate whether people are unequally located in the social structure as a result of structures which systematically advantage some groups and disadvantage others. Evidence is needed, too, that people's unequal social positions underlie their unequal health. As Fabienne Peter notes, 'to be able to pass a judgement on social inequalities in health, we need an understanding of the underlying causes' (2004: 104).

If understandings of causes are required to pass judgement on health inequalities, then social and health research has a critical role to play in reaching conclusions about health equity and social justice. Such research has a key role to play too, in informing policies to support greater equality in people's basic freedoms, including their opportunities for health (see Box 1.11). *Unequal Lives* makes a contribution to the research task. The chapters which follow provide insights into the patterns and causes of socio-economic inequalities and the pathways through which they shape people's health.

---

**Box 1.11**

'[T]o act justly in health policy, we must have knowledge about the causal pathways through which socioeconomic (and other) inequalities work to produce differential health outcomes.' (Daniels *et al.*, 2004: 79)

---

# 2 Measuring health and health inequalities

## 2.1 Introduction

Life expectancy in the UK reached 50 years in the early twentieth century (Whitehead, 1997). A hundred years on, life expectancy has yet to pass the 50-year threshold in the world's poorest countries (Goesling and Firebaugh, 2004). It is therefore not surprising that survival continues to be the major indicator of people's health, with the health of nations measured by how long people live and how many of them die each year. Data on length of life and rates of death are combined with information on people's socio-economic circumstances to map inequalities in their health.

But, of course, mortality-based statistics are based on information about those who died. They do not directly capture the health of people who stay alive. A significant proportion will have health problems which, while carrying a low mortality risk, are chronic and debilitating. Data on mortality and life expectancy are therefore increasingly supplemented by information on the health of the living. Important among these measures are subjective assessments of health status as well as those which capture the process of health development and decline across the life course.

Whatever measures are used to assess people's health, health researchers need information about the population in order to estimate the proportion in poor health. For countries which undertake a regular census of the population, this provides the key data source. In the UK, census-based data are adjusted for under-enumeration. Crude (actual) rates of ill health and death can also be adjusted to take account of the sex and age structure of the population: for example, to take account of a higher than average proportion of older people in some areas. There are agreed procedures for doing this: for 'standardizing' for differences in the composition of study populations. Age-standardized rates estimate what the crude rate would have been if the population had had a similar age structure to an agreed standard population. One widely used standard is the European standard population, constructed by the WHO for standardizing health data between European countries.

The first part of the chapter discusses key indicators of health. Sections 2.2 to 2.4 look in turn at measures based on mortality, on people's assessments of their current health status and on people's broader health trajectories. The chapter also briefly considers the measurement of health inequalities, noting the important distinction between absolute and relative measures of inequality. More detailed reviews of the measurement of health and health inequalities are available elsewhere (see Wagstaff *et al.*, 1991; Manor *et al.*, 1997; Bhopal, 2002; Bowling, 2002). The aim here is to introduce measures which are widely used in health inequalities research – and therefore in the chapters which follow.

## 2.2 Measuring health: mortality-based measures

### Mortality rates

Information on the number and causes of death has long been used to measure the health of populations. Such information has been routinely collected in Britain since the sixteenth century. The early data collection systems were locally based, with parish records providing details of deaths and burials. Figure 2.1 gives an example of these Bills of Mortality for London for a week in 1665, the year in which the Great Plague struck the city's population. As it indicates, around 8000 burials were recorded, with deaths from causes ranging from 'aged' through 'griping in the guts' and 'teeth' to 'wormes'. But dominating the mortality statistics is the bubonic plague, which accounted for over 85 per cent of deaths.

By the mid-nineteenth century, England and Wales had both a national system of registration for births and deaths, and a schema for classifying cause of death. This schema, in turn, formed the basis of the International Classification of Disease (ICD). Established in 1900, ICD–1 had fewer than 200 codes for different causes of death (but none for wormes!). The ICD has been repeatedly updated to take account of advances in medical knowledge and the emergence of new diseases: lung cancer, for example, did not have its own code until 1940 (Griffiths and Brock, 2003). Its current revision, ICD–10, has over 5000 codes.

The ICD groups diseases and injuries into broad categories, like diseases of the circulatory system, diseases of the respiratory system and neoplasms (cancer), with each category containing a set of more precise diagnostic codes. For example, hypertension, ischemic heart disease and cerebrovascular disease (of which stroke is the major type) have codes within the category of circulatory disease, and influenza and pneumonia within the category of respiratory disease (WHO, 1992).

## The Diseases and Casualties this Week.

| | |
|---|---|
| Imposthume | 11 |
| Infants | 16 |
| Killed by a fall from the Belfrey at Alhallows the Great | 1 |
| Kingsevil | 2 |
| Lethargy | 1 |
| Palsie | 1 |
| Plague | 7165 |
| A Bortive | 5 |
| Aged | 43 |
| Ague | 2 |
| Apoplexie | 1 |
| Bleeding | 2 |
| Rickets | 17 |
| Rising of the Lights | 11 |
| Scowring | 5 |
| Scurvy | 2 |
| Spleen | 1 |
| Burnt in his Bed by a Candle at St. Giles Cripplegate | 1 |
| Spotted Feaver | 101 |
| Stilborn | 17 |
| Canker | 1 |
| Childbed | 42 |
| Chrisomes | 18 |
| Consumption | 134 |
| Convulsion | 64 |
| Cough | 2 |
| Dropsie | 33 |
| Feaver | 309 |
| Stone | 2 |
| Stopping of the stomach | 9 |
| Strangury | 1 |
| Suddenly | 1 |
| Surfeit | 49 |
| Teeth | 121 |
| Thrush | 5 |
| Timpany | 1 |
| Flox and Small-pox | 5 |
| Frighted | 3 |
| Gowt | 1 |
| Grief | 3 |
| Griping in the Guts | 51 |
| Jaundies | 5 |
| Tissick | 11 |
| Vomiting | 3 |
| Winde | 3 |
| Wormes | 15 |

Christned ⎨ Males — 95, Females — 81, In all — 176 ⎬   Buried ⎨ Males — 4095, Females — 4202, In all — 8297 ⎬ Plague — 7165

Increased in the Burials this Week — 607

Parishes clear of the Plague — 4    Parishes Infected — 126

The Assize of Bread set forth by Order of the Lord Maior and Court of Aldermen; A penny Wheaten Loaf to contain Nine Ounces and a half, and three half-penny White Loaves the like weight.

**Figure 2.1**  Bills of Mortality for London for one week, 1665

*Source:* Museum of London. Reproduced under licence and with permission of the Museum of London Picture Library

Using ICD–10, deaths are attributed to a single underlying cause. This underlying cause is the disease or injury which resulted in death. Expressed more formally, 'the underlying cause of death is (a) the disease or injury that initiated the train of events leading to death or (b) the circumstances of the accident or violence which produced the fatal injury' (WHO, 1977: 763). For most causes of death in the UK, an underlying cause is assigned through an automated coding system from information recorded on coroner certificates. The coding process indicates that the ICD–10 categories of circulatory disease, cancer and respiratory disease are the major causes of death, and together account for 77 per cent of deaths in England and Wales in 2005 (Health Statistics Quarterly, 2006a). Table 2.1 moves beyond these broad categories to give details of the leading causes of death in England and Wales. The league table is led by two circulatory diseases: ischemic heart disease and cerebro-vascular disease. Also known as coronary artery disease, ischemic heart disease is a condition where narrowed or blocked blood vessels affect the supply of blood to the heart, thus reducing or cutting off the supply of oxygen and nutrients that it needs. Cerebrovascular disease affects the blood vessels of the brain (or vessels supplying the brain); stroke is the major, but not only, example. Cancer (neoplasms) of the trachea, bronchus and lung is the leading cause of cancer deaths.

**Table 2.1**   Leading causes of death by sex, 2005, England and Wales

| Underlying cause | % of all deaths | Age-standardized rate per 100,000 population |
|---|---|---|
| *Men* | | |
| 1. Ischemic heart disease | 20.2 | 146.2 |
| 2. Cerebrovascular disease | 7.9 | 55.1 |
| 3. Malignant neoplasm of trachea, bronchus and lung | 6.9 | 51.1 |
| 4. Chronic lower respiratory disease | 5.6 | 38.9 |
| 5. Influenza and pneumonia | 5.0 | 35.3 |
| 6. Malignant neoplasm of prostate | 3.7 | 25.5 |
| *Women* | | |
| 1. Ischemic heart disease | 14.5 | 68.5 |
| 2. Cerebrovascular disease | 11.7 | 51.8 |
| 3. Influenza and pneumonia | 7.7 | 29.8 |
| 4. Dementia and alzheimer's disease | 4.8 | 18.7 |
| 5. Chronic lower respiratory disease | 4.7 | 25.1 |
| 6. Malignant neoplasm of trachea, bronchus and lung | 4.4 | 28.9 |

Reproduced under the terms of the click-use licence.

*Source:* Health Statistics Quarterly (2006b)

The recording practices through which mortality data are generated need to be born in mind when interpreting such statistics. First, changes to the ICD can change the cause to which deaths are assigned. For instance, the introduction of the new ICD–10 has had the effect of taking a significant proportion of deaths out of the respiratory disease category, resulting in a 22 per cent reduction in deaths from this cause (Brock *et al.*, 2006). As this suggests, the century-long process of revision makes it difficult to measure historical trends in specific causes with precision. Second, the coding procedures mean that some diseases and circumstances are more likely to be identified as the underlying cause than others. When death certificates record major cardiovascular events, like stroke or myocardial infarction, and major cancers, like lung cancer, they are almost always defined as 'the disease which initiated the train of events leading to death'. In contrast, diabetes is rarely given as the underlying cause of death, figuring instead as contributing to death by compromising survival from other conditions (Devis and Rooney, 1999). The question of what constitutes the underlying cause has relevance beyond high-income countries like the UK. In low-income countries, the underlying cause of many childhood deaths is recorded as infectious disease. But malnutrition reduces the body's defences against disease – and inadequate food supplies, poor sanitation and unsafe water sources increase the risk of malnutrition. Third, nationally and internationally, deaths resulting from war are not systematically included in the death registration process and are therefore often missing from cause of death data (Lopez *et al.*, 2006). In the UK context, deaths in the armed forces overseas are not included in mortality statistics.

## Life expectancy

Death rates are used to calculate life expectancy, the most widely used indicator of population health. Life expectancy at birth estimates the average number of years a newborn baby can expect to live, if the patterns of mortality at the time of their birth were to stay the same throughout their life. Deaths in the first year of life have the largest impact on average life expectancy, with deaths at older ages having progressively less effect on overall life expectancy. To provide a measure of health at older ages, life expectancy at age 65 estimates the number of years that a person who survives to this age can expect to live. Life expectancies at birth and at age 65 are given for the UK in Box 2.1.

In countries where many children die (and life expectancy is therefore low), deaths in early life provide a sensitive measure of people's health. Thus in nineteenth- and early twentieth-century Britain, infant mortality (deaths in the first year of life) and deaths among children under the age of 5 (under-5 mortality) were widely used measures of health. In 1911, for example, more than one child in ten died before their first birthday (Registrar General, 1913).

---

**Box 2.1 Life expectancy**

In the UK in 2002:

life expectancy at birth reached 75.9 for men and 80.5 for women. In recent decades, the rate of increase has been faster for men than for women.
life expectancy at age 65 stood at 16.1 years for men and 19.1 years for women. (Health Statistics Quarterly, 2006b)

---

A century later, infant morality and under-5 mortality capture the scale of global health inequalities. In high-income countries, around 7 in every 1000 children die before they reach the age of 5; in low-income countries, over 120 children in every 1000 do not reach their fifth birthday (World Bank, 2003).

As death rates have fallen and life expectancy has risen, health researchers have increasingly looked beyond measures of survival to measures of health. They have looked, in particular, to measures which give people an opportunity to assess their own health.

## 2.3 Measuring health: measures based on people's assessment of their health status

Examples of measures which seek to capture people's subjective health status include *self-assessed health*, based on rating scales provided by the researcher, and *limiting long-standing illness*, based on people's answers to questions about health conditions which restrict their everyday activities. Questions relating to these two dimensions are routinely asked in UK health surveys; in 2001, both were included in the decennial Census.

Self-assessed health provides an overall measure of health, with the respondent invited to rate their health using a preset rating scale. Examples for the UK are given in Box 2.2. While the scales can be criticized for being prescriptive, the data they generate provide a broad indication of people's subjective health status. They suggest that a significant minority, rate their health as less than good (see Figure 1.1) and that the proportion increases in line with increasing social disadvantage (Figure 1.2). Such information is important in its own right, as a measure of how healthy people feel themselves to be. In addition, self-assessed health is an accurate predictor of an individual's future risk of death. In follow-up studies, people who assessed their health as poor had higher death rates than those who rated their health more positively. This predictive effect remains when other measures of health status are included in the analysis, like nurse-performed assessments, information

---

**Box 2.2 Questions on self-assessed health asked in key UK health surveys**

---

*General Household Survey (Britain), Continuous Health Survey (Northern Ireland), UK Census*
    'Over the last 12 months would you say your health has on the whole been good, fairly good, or not good?'

*Health Survey for England, Scottish Health Survey*
    'How is your health in general? Would you say it is very good, good, fair, bad, very bad?'

---

from medical records and measures of chronic conditions. As the authors of a major review conclude, 'self-ratings of health, which take only seconds to obtain in a survey interview, reliably predict survival in populations even when known health risk factors have been accounted for' (Idler and Benyamini, 1997: 26).

Combining information on life expectancy and self-assessed health provides estimates of how long people can expect to live in good health. In the UK, estimates have been derived from the proportion of people assessing their health as 'not good' in health surveys and the 2001 Census, with the latter used to extend coverage to residents of communal establishments (Breakwell and Bajekal, 2006). Called health expectancy, healthy life expectancy or health-adjusted life expectancy, estimates measure expected years of healthy life. Health expectancy is considerably shorter than life expectancy; the gender gap in health expectancy is also considerably smaller (Box 2.3).

A second widely used measure of overall health status is derived from information on long-term illnesses. Major health surveys typically use a two-stage question which asks everyone about long-standing conditions, and then asks those who report them whether the conditions impose restrictions on their activities (Box 2.4). A shortened version is now included in the UK Census (Box 2.4). Answers to these questions suggest that around 1 in 5 adults in Britain have one or more long-term conditions which restrict their activity;

---

**Box 2.3 Health expectancy**

---

In the UK in 2002:
        men could expect to live 75.9 years and 67.1 years in good health
        women could expect to live 80.5 years and 69.9 years in good health.
(Health Statistics Quarterly, 2006b)

---

**Box 2.4 Limiting long-term illness**

---

*General Household Survey (Britain), Health Survey for England, Continuous Health Survey (Northern Ireland), Scottish Health Survey*
   'Do you have any long-standing illness, disability or infirmity? By long-standing I mean anything that has troubled you over period of time or that is likely to affect you over a period of time? Yes/no
   If yes: does this illness or disability/do any of these illnesses or disabilities limit your activities in any way? Yes/no'

*UK Census 2001*
   'Do you have any long-standing illness, disability or infirmity which limits your daily activities or the work you can do? Yes/no'

---

among those aged 50 and over, the proportion rises to 1 in 3 (ONS, 2001; McMunn *et al.*, 2003). Among older people, the most frequently reported chronic conditions relate to the musculoskeletal system (the system of bones, muscles and joints which gives people the ability to stand and move) and the cardiovascular system (the system that circulates blood through the body, including the heart, blood and blood vessels).

Limiting long-term illness often serves as a measure of disability, with information used to derive estimates of expected years of life without disability (called 'disability-free life expectancy'). It is a measure which captures the prevalence of chronic and debilitating conditions. For example, UK estimates suggest that men can expect to spend 15 years of their life living with an illness or impairment which restricts their everyday activities, a period which represents 20 per cent of their total life span. At age 65, they can expect to spend over half their remaining years with a limiting condition (Health Statistics Quarterly, 2006b). Women can anticipate spending more of their lives, both in years and as a proportion of their expected lifespan, with a condition which, in Sen's terms, constrains what they can do and be (see Chapter 1, section 1.3 for a discussion of Sen's capability perspective).

While such information provides an insight into the quality of people's health, it derives from an approach to defining and measuring disability which has been heavily criticized. For over 30 years, disability researchers and activists have argued against the assumptions which underpin questions like those in Box 2.4 (see, for example, Abberley, 1990; Oliver, 1996; Thomas, 1999). They point out that the questions are framed in ways which imply that restrictions of activity are caused by, and are inherent properties of, the long-standing condition. In other words, it is the 'long-standing illness, disability or infirmity' which is seen to be limiting, not the circumstances in which it is experienced. Disability studies, and the disability movement more

broadly, reject this perspective. They point out that the major cause of limitations associated with chronic illness and impairment are socially imposed
barriers: the disabling nature of the built environment, prejudicial attitudes
and discriminatory practices at school and in the workplace (Campbell and
Oliver, 1996). It is a perspective which emphasizes the socially contingent
nature of disability: when barriers are reduced, so too are the restrictions of
activity. Box 2.5, taken from a letter included in Carol Thomas's book on
women's experiences of disability, provides a glimpse into what reducing
barriers means.

This social model of disability, as it is called, is increasingly understood
and accepted: it has, for example, informed the new *International Classification
of Functioning, Disability and Health* (WHO, 2001). The model uses the twin
terms of impairment and disability to capture the distinction between functional limitations and environmental restrictions. As Box 2.6 indicates,
*impairment* refers to restrictions related to illness or injury; *disability* to restrictions which result from the exclusionary practices of the wider society. For
example, a stroke or a spinal injury may impair people's physical mobility;

---

**Box 2.5**

'Lisa, a wheelchair user in her mid-twenties at the time of writing. (Extracts from
her letter.)

When I first left the spinal (injury) unit at 19 years of age I had to rely very heavily
on my family. At my parents' home there were no facilities for me (bathroom
and toilet). So for several months I had a commode and bed baths in my Mum's
front room . . . The worst thing about those first few months at home was having
to rely on everyone to drive me from A to B. Now seven years down the road,
I have my own one bedroom adapted flat . . . I work full-time . . . and I drive
my own hand controlled car. It's been a struggle to get completely independent but it's worth it, and I wouldn't give it up for anyone.' (Quoted in Thomas,
1999: 18)

---

**Box 2.6**

'*Impairment* is the functional limitation within the individual caused by physical,
mental or sensory impairment.
*Disability* is the loss or limitation of opportunities to take part in the normal
life of the community on an equal basis with others due to physical and social
barriers'. (UPIAS, 1976: 3–4, cited in Bickenbach *et al.*, 1999: 1176)

these impairments become disabilities when people who use mobility aids, like sticks and wheelchairs, find their way blocked – often literally – to places and opportunities which non-disabled people can take for granted. It is a perspective which suggests that statistics generated from questions like those in Box 2.4 conflate the distinction which is central to people's experiences, and the wider politics, of disability. As a result, 'disability statistics' typically measure the number of people experiencing limitations of activity resulting from the combined effects of impairment and disability. Such statistics need to be interpreted with this in mind.

An appreciation that the experience of limiting long-term illness is socially mediated, highlights a more general feature of subjective measures of health. The meanings of categories, like good health and limiting illness, which underpin such measures are likely to change as individuals get older and their circumstances become more (or less) restricting. At the societal level, meanings may also change, with increasing life expectancy and advances in medical care raising people's expectations for their health. This suggests that caution should be exercised when comparing patterns of self-assessed health and limiting illness over time and between societies.

## 2.4 Measuring health: measures of development and decline

Traditional indicators of health provide a snapshot of people's health at particular points in time. Mortality-based measures capture health at the end of life, recording the fact and cause of death. Health surveys, too, tend to focus on a relatively narrow time window, asking people to reflect on how they currently feel about their health and about limitations that their health may impose on their activity.

This approach is being supplemented by one which takes a more dynamic view of health. Its concern is with how health develops and declines across the life course. It therefore puts less emphasis on health status – on self-assessed health, limiting illnesses and death – and more on the developmental and degenerative processes associated with the journey from 'womb to tomb'. While much is still to be uncovered about these processes, it is clear that they are characterized by rapid development in the early years of life, a peak or plateau in adulthood, and decline through middle and old age (Kuh and Ben-Shlomo, 2004). For example, muscle strength typically increases rapidly through childhood and into early adulthood, and then declines from midlife, a decline that is an important contributor to physical frailty among older people (Aihie Sayer and Cooper, 2004). Studies are highlighting similar trajectories of development and decline for cognition, a term that describes mental functions like the ability to think, learn, reason and remember.

Cognitive skills, as measured by attention span, verbal skills, problem-solving and memory, develop very rapidly in the first few years of life, reach a plateau in early adulthood before starting to decline.

New concepts and measures are being introduced to capture these health trajectories. Two examples are given here, relating respectively to the early years of life and to midlife and older age.

For the early years, the concept of *developmental health* has been proposed (Keating and Hertzman, 1999). The concept captures the fact that health in childhood is 'underdevelopment', a development integral to the process of growth and maturation which mark a child's journey from birth, through infancy and later childhood, and into adolescence. The concept is multi-dimensional, embracing physical and emotional development as well as the development of cognitive and social skills. Measures of developmental health include indicators of physical growth before and after birth, like birth weight and rate of growth in childhood, as well as cognitive ability (for example, verbal ability, numeracy and literacy skills) and emotional well-being (for example, self-esteem).

For midlife and older age, attention shifts from the development to the maintenance of bodily functions. Studies in the UK suggest that the majority of older people are positive about the experience of ageing, and continue to be so up to and beyond the age of 85 (Demakakos *et al.*, 2006). Nonetheless, getting older is associated with changes in body systems and capacities. A range of concepts are used to describe this process, including *functional ageing*. The concept draws attention to the functioning of body systems, like the musculo-skeletal and cardiovascular systems. The concept, therefore has some parallels with the concept of impairment (Box 2.6), casting impairment as a dynamic process in which limitations of function develop and intensify as the body ages. Figure 2.2 captures this process for physical impairment in a large survey of older people, the *English Longitudinal Study of Ageing* (Melzer *et al.*, 2006). It is based on a widely used measure of impairment, called the Short Physical Performance Battery, which combines three dimensions of physical function-ing into a single score. The dimensions are standing up from a sitting position, balance when standing and walking speed. Figure 2.2 describes the proportion of men and women with poor physical functioning, a measure of health which predicts future disease, disability and mortality (Aihie Sayer and Cooper, 2004; Power and Kuh, 2006). As Figure 2.2 indicates, levels of physical impairment increase markedly with age, with the rate of increase more marked among women than men.

Studies which follow-up children through their lives are the key resource for understanding developmental health and functional ageing. They are pointing to the links between health in early and later life, with the health reserves accumulated through childhood having a lasting influence on health in adulthood. As the evidence discussed in Chapter 10 suggests, inequalities

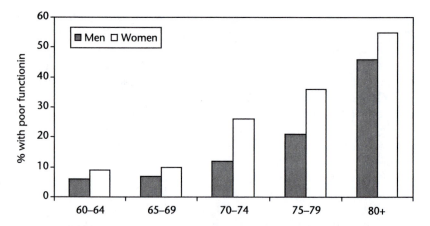

**Figure 2.2** Physical impairment as measured by the Short Physical Performance Battery (score ≤ 8) among adults aged 60 years and over, England, 2004–5

*Source:* adapted from Melzer *et al.*, 2006, table 6A.9

in children's environments can become embedded in patterns of development in ways which have lifelong effects on health.

## 2.5 Measuring health inequalities

As noted in Chapter 1, health inequity is seen as a normative concept. Health inequities can therefore not be directly measured. What are measured are health inequalities. Socio-economic inequalities are captured in a range of indicators of socio-economic position, like occupational status and income (discussed in Chapter 4, section 4.3). As later chapters note, these indicators reveal inequalities in all the dimensions of health discussed in this chapter: for traditional measures, like mortality and life expectancy, subjective measures of health, like self-assessed health and limiting long-term illness, as well as for measures of health development and decline.

For some health outcomes and for some age and gender groups, health inequalities take the form of a steady gradient, with each step down the socio-economic ladder bringing a stepped increase in the prevalence of poor health. An example is given in Figure 2.3. It focuses on ischemic heart disease, the leading cause of death among men and women in the UK, and plots the rates among men aged 35–64 by social class (White *et al.*, 2003). The social class classification, described in more detail in Chapter 4, section 4.3, is based on occupation and runs from professional and managerial (social class I and II) through skilled non-manual and skilled manual (IIINM and IIIM), to semi-skilled and unskilled manual (IV and V).

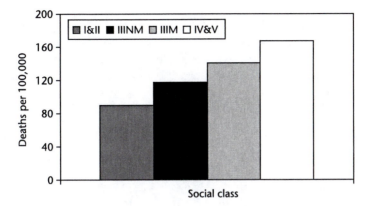

**Figure 2.3**   Deaths from ischemic heart disease by social class, men aged 35–64, England and Wales, 1997–9 (age-standardized death rates per 100,000 person years)

*Source:* adapted from White *et al.*, 2003, table 3

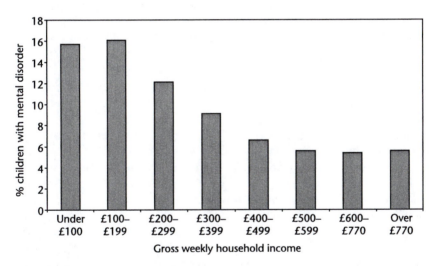

**Figure 2.4**   Prevalence of mental disorder in children aged 5–15 by gross weekly household income, Britain, 1999

*Source:* adapted from Melzer and Gatwood, 2000, table 4.8

Health inequalities do not always take a monotonic form. For example, in some instances, the gradient flattens out at the higher and/or lower ends of the socio-economic hierarchy. Figure 2.4 illustrates this pattern. It maps the rates of mental disorder among children in richer and poorer households in Britain in the late 1990s. It is based on data collected from children, parents and teachers in a study which focused on emotional, hyperactivity and conduct disorders suffered to a degree which was distressing and interfered with children's lives (Meltzer and Gatwood, 2000). Rather than a stepwise relationship between income level and rate of mental disorder across the whole income distribution, Figure 2.4 points to a 'threshold effect' at both the higher and lower ends. Above a threshold of £500 a week, increases in incomes are not associated with further declines in rates of mental disorders; below a threshold of £200 a week, there is a sharp increase in the rate, with no further rise for the lowest-income group. Like stepwise gradients, threshold patterns can change over time. In a more recent survey of children's mental health, a more complex pattern emerges and the low-income threshold extends further up the income distribution (Green *et al.*, 2005).

The inequalities captured in Figures 2.3 and 2.4 can be represented in different ways. An important distinction is between absolute and relative measures of health inequalities. Both typically take the most advantaged group as the reference group, and compare the health of other groups against the standard achieved by this reference group.

*Absolute differences* are the differences in the rates of ill health: for instance, the difference in rates of premature death in more and less advantaged groups. Death rates from ischemic heart disease provide an example (Figure 2.3). Among men aged 35–64, rates stood at 167 per 100,000 in social class IV and V (semi-skilled and unskilled manual) and 90 in social class I and II (professional and managerial). The absolute difference was therefore 77 deaths per 100,000 (167 deaths per 100,000 minus 90 deaths per 100,000).

*Relative differences* take these health data and present them in a way which tells us how much more likely poorer groups are to experience the health problem than better-off groups. Taking the example of heart disease again, a quick 'eye-balling' of Figure 2.3 suggests that the risk of death from ischemic heart disease for men in the poorest circumstances is nearly twice that of men in the most advantaged positions. Their risk is in fact 1.86 times greater, a risk ratio calculated by dividing 167 by 90. Put the other way around, relative measures indicate how much better the health chances of privileged groups are than those in poorer circumstances. With respect to heart disease, again, the risk of death for a man at the top of the social class ladder is half (.54) that of a man at the bottom of the ladder (a risk ratio calculated by dividing 90 by 167).

Another example may help to illustrate these two ways of measuring health inequalities. The illustration is provided by infant mortality, a key marker of both child and population health, and one for which there is good historical data (Table 2.2). In England and Wales in 1911, infant mortality rates stood at 152.4 per 1000 among children born to fathers in unskilled manual occupations (social class V) and 76.4 per 1000 among children born to professional parents (social class I): an absolute difference

**Table 2.2**   Infant mortality (deaths per 1000 live births) in social class I and V in 1911 and 2001, England and Wales

|  | Social class I | Social class V | Absolute inequalities | Relative inequalities |
|---|---|---|---|---|
| 1911 | 76.4 | 152.4 | 76.0 deaths per 1000 (152.4 − 76.4 = 76.0) | 2.00 × risk of death (152.4/76.4 = 2.0) |
| 2001 | 3.8 | 7.4 | 3.6 deaths per 1000 (7.4 − 3.8 = 3.6) | 1.95 × risk of death (7.4/3.8 = 1.95) |

*Source:* adapted from Registrar General (1913) (1911 data); Rowan (2003: table 5) (2001 data)

in death rates of 76.0 deaths per year (Registrar General, 1913). These large absolute differences were matched by large relative differences in the risk of death: children born to parents at the bottom of the class hierarchy were twice as likely to die before their first birthday as children born to parents at the top (152.4 divided by 76.4). Changes in the occupational classification means that class inequalities across the twentieth century cannot be strictly compared. Nonetheless, data for 2001 point to a dramatic reduction in death rates in the first year of life for children in social class I and V. Rates in 2001 stood at 3.8 and 7.4 per 1000 respectively (Rowan, 2003). Absolute differences in death rates had therefore fallen between 1911 and 2001 from 76.0 per 1000 (152.4 minus 76.4) to 3.6 per 1000 (7.4 minus 3.8). But while absolute inequalities had narrowed, relative inequalities were unchanged. In 2001, as in 1911, the odds of death were still twice as high for children born into the poorest circumstances.

Both absolute and relative differences provide summary measures of the scale of health inequalities. Both are therefore important when describing inequalities at particular points in time. However, relative measures are widely regarded as more appropriate for tracking changes in health inequalities over time, particularly when overall levels of health are rising (Victora *et al.*, 2000). This is because, as health improves, absolute differences tend to narrow: there are fewer deaths in all groups and therefore the absolute differences between them become smaller. Relative measures take the baseline level of health into account. They calculate rates in one group as a proportion of rates in the reference group.

Whether absolute or relative measures of health inequalities are used, the focus is typically on the gap between groups at the extreme ends of the hierarchy. For example, in the examples of infant mortality given above, the comparison is between children in the most and least privileged class groups. The advantaged group is typically the reference category against which the poorest group is compared: for example, 'rates of x (the outcome under investigation) are twice as high in the lowest as highest social class'. It is a way of representing health inequalities which is widely used in research and policy. It succinctly conveys the magnitude of social and health inequalities, as illustrated by the examples given for infant mortality rates and premature death rates from ischemic heart disease. However, as with all statistics, attention needs to be given to their interpretation. Three points should be borne in mind throughout the chapters which follow.

First, what begins as a statistical comparison can quickly become a normative comparison, with the lives and lifestyles of poorer groups and communities judged against those of the best-off. Viewed in this way, lifestyle differences – higher rates of teenage motherhood, for example, or higher rates of cigarette smoking – can be seen as cultural deficits. In other words, researchers and policy-makers focus on what poorer groups lack, not on the privileges which richer groups enjoy. Second, knowing that the risk of an adverse outcome is greater for a poorer child than for a child from a more privileged background does not tell us how likely it is. To know how likely it is, we need to know how many children experience it. In the example of infant mortality, 1 in 135 (7.4 in 1000) children in social class V die in the first year of life. In other words, while the relative risk of death is much higher for poorer children than it is for their more advantaged peers, death rates among poor children in the UK, as in other high-income countries, are low. Third, the focus on the top and bottom of the social hierarchy means that nothing is revealed about the intermediate groups which lie between them. In the UK, these intermediate groups constitute 90 per cent of the population: social class I and V make up respectively 5 per cent and 6 per cent of the adult population (ONS, 2001). It is important to remember that, across these groups, health continues to be patterned by socio-economic position.

## 2.6 Conclusions

The chapter has provided a brief overview of measures of health. It has included established measures, like death rates, life expectancy and self-assessed health. It has discussed, too, measures which take a more dynamic approach to health and seek to capture its development in childhood and its maintenance and decline in middle and older age. Each of these measures point to marked socio-economic inequalities in health.

These inequalities can be expressed as absolute and relative differences. Whichever metric is chosen, people in the most advantaged circumstances are often taken as the reference group. Standards in the poorest countries and communities are compared against those achieved by the richest ones. Setting the benchmark in this way has considerable appeal. It captures the fact and magnitude of health inequalities. It also rightly puts the focus on levelling up and not levelling down: on raising the level of health in poorer groups closer to that enjoyed by the most advantaged groups. But there are drawbacks to defining the advantaged group as the reference case. It becomes the normative group whose living circumstances and lifestyles are not held up for scrutiny: the spotlight is turned, instead, on the lives of the poor. In the chapters which follow, there is dual focus on both privilege and poverty, and on the mechanisms through which both are sustained.

# 3 Socio-economic inequalities

## 3.1 Introduction

Health researchers use a range of measures of socio-economic position to map the association between people's unequal lives and their unequal health. The figures in Chapters 1 and 2, for example, were based on own occupation and household income. Because they measure it at these micro levels, health researchers tend to regard socio-economic position as a property of individuals and families. It is something people have, like a high educational qualification, a high-status job or a high income. Gender and ethnicity tend to be treated in the same way, as personal characteristics and individual variables.

Social researchers have a different way of seeing people's social position. Their perspectives are informed by sociology and social policy, disciplines which look outward from the individual to the society of which they are part. Socio-economic position, like other social positions, are therefore regarded less as stable attributes of individuals and more as dynamic elements of social structures. It is a perspective which provides rich insights into the mechanisms through which social inequalities are produced and reproduced over time.

Sociological perspectives on socio-economic position emphasize its double sided quality. It is a social location into which people are slotted – and one which people actively construct for themselves. In other words, socio-economic position is both structurally imposed and socially produced, with the resulting inequalities in people's positions woven into the fabric of their daily lives. Sections 3.3 and 3.4 explore these dual dimensions. Section 3.2 sets the scene by briefly discussing the changing fortunes of research on socio-economic inequality in sociology and social policy. In both disciplines, 'social class' and 'class inequality' tend to be preferred to 'socio-economic position' and 'socio-economic inequality', the terms more commonly found in health research. Positioned at the interface of social and health research, the chapter, like the book as a whole, therefore moves between these different vocabularies. It treats the concepts of social class and socio-economic position as equivalent and the terms, therefore, as interchangeable.

## 3.2 Researching socio-economic inequalities

The origins of sociology and social policy lie in the social and economic changes associated with the industrialization of northern Europe and North America in the nineteenth and early twentieth centuries. It was a process in which agriculture gave way to industry as the source of national wealth, and manufacturing became a major source of employment. 'Industrial societies' was the term coined for societies whose economic base lay in mining and manufacturing. While the new systems of production created jobs and fuelled economic growth, the early social scientists found that inequalities remained entrenched and pervasive. This conclusion was most forcefully expressed by Karl Marx. He argued that, far from softening social inequalities, the emerging capitalist systems of production were hardening and intensifying the age-old division between 'exploited and exploiting, dominated and dominating' (Marx and Engels, 1888: 13).

Like Marx and Engels, early social researchers focused on inequalities linked to what people owned and how they earned their living. It was a focus crystallized in the concept of social class, a concept which played a formative role in the twentieth-century history of the disciplines of sociology and social policy in Britain (Savage, 2000). But through the 1980s and 1990s, the concept lost its central position (Skeggs, 1997; Savage, 2000). It was knocked from its perch by a series of influential critiques which, while their lines of attack varied, concluded that 'class is an outmoded concept' (Clark and Lipset, 1991: 397).

The conclusion is based on two related lines of argument. First, a concept developed to make sense of the social order created through the process of industrialization is seen to give little analytic purchase on societies whose economies are no longer dominated by industries like mining, steel and manufacturing. Instead of the industrial sector, it is the service sector, and particularly business and financial services, which are the engine of economic growth. 'Industrial society', a construct built around mass production, manual work and male breadwinners, is therefore being replaced by a new set of descriptors, including 'advanced capitalist societies' and 'post-industrial societies'.

Second, changes in the labour market are being accompanied by the emergence of new patterns of family life and community allegiance which are transforming the social structure which once typified the UK and other older industrial countries. These transformations are seen as part of a broader fracturing of social hierarchies – a fracturing in which people are breaking free not only from their class positions but from those grounded in gender, ethnicity and sexuality. Released from the grip of these multiple structures of inequality, people are seen as self-fashioning their lives: crafting identities and constructing lifestyles which express their unique individuality. In this new social landscape, it is not people's position in the labour market – as employers and employees, exploiters and exploited – which matters. Instead, social differentiation is seen to be based on people's position as consumers, with people expressing their individuality through how they spend their money and what they do in their leisure time (Box 3.1). In this consumption-oriented world, it is argued that inequalities of the workplace no longer dominate people's destinies. Concepts like social class are therefore redundant as tools of social analysis.

While such arguments had a powerful hold on sociological debates of the 1980s and 1990s, they are being increasingly challenged. The conclusion that the concept of social class has outlived its usefulness is being questioned on both empirical and theoretical grounds.

The empirical challenge comes primarily from the discipline of social policy, a discipline which maintained its focus on social class across decades in which the concept faded from view in sociology. Studies in the UK have uncovered little evidence that socio-economic inequalities are withering away. They suggest instead that they have become more entrenched, with the proceeds of economic growth disproportionately going to those who are already well-off (Goodman and Shepherd, 2002; Brewer *et al.*, 2006). As a result, the richest 10 per cent of the population own well over 50 per cent of the country's marketable wealth (Hills, 2004). Similarly, recent decades have seen both the persistence and the widening of educational inequalities, with the children of poorer parents in manual occupations deriving much less benefit from society's investment in the expansion of higher education than children of richer parents in professional occupations (Machin and Vignoles, 2004; Blanden *et al.*, 2005). Taken together, empirical studies provide little support for the view that

---

**Box 3.1**

'The economic trends of the post-war world have been seen as undermining the conditions which gave rise to class relations in modernity as part of a shift from production to a new era of "post-modernity" based on consumption. As the workplace and economic relations which once defined "class" societies have been eclipsed by the increasing centrality of consumption, so class allegiances have been replaced by . . . consumption differences which produce a kaleidoscope of lifestyles, rather than distinct social class divisions.' (Bottero, 2005: 128)

social class in the UK is losing its influence on people's lives. Evidence from other high-income countries, too, gives little ground for believing that people's labour market position and economic resources no longer matter (see, for example, Mishel *et al.*, 2006, on the USA and Palme *et al.*, 2003, on Sweden).

The theoretical challenge builds on this evidence. It argues that social class still has a powerful hold on people's lives, but the processes through which it operates are changing. While occupation is still central, non-economic assets are identified as increasingly important in maintaining people's advantaged positions. These non-economic assets include styles of speech, dress and social interaction – with employers seen to attach greater importance to such markers of social background than they did in the past.

Summarizing this empirical and theoretical literature is no easy task. There is a voluminous literature and the theoretical debates are often couched in an opaque language hard to fathom for those not schooled in sociology and cultural studies (and perhaps even for those who are!). Identifying overarching themes inevitably means reducing the richness and obscuring the disagreements which are the hallmark of much sociological analysis. Two broad and enduring themes nonetheless stand out.

The first theme suggests that an individual's socio-economic position is shaped by unequal structures which exist outside their lives. It therefore lays stress on socio-economic positions as *structural locations*, as tightly regulated places in the social hierarchy. The second theme suggests that socio-economic positions are *actively produced* and reproduced by people going about their lives. The themes are, of course, two sides of a single coin: individuals are constrained by their position in the social hierarchy which, at the same time, is sustained by their actions. It is a coin whose sides carry the twinned concepts of 'structure' and 'agency', concepts which have long run through sociological debates about inequality (see Bottero, 2005, for an overview). It is as a two-sided coin captured, too, in Marx's dictum that people make their own histories but not in circumstances of their choosing (Box 3.2). This means that external circumstances and self-made histories are inseparable aspects of inequality and inseparable aspects of daily life. But distinguishing between them can help to see that inequality has multiple dimensions. Sections 3.3 and 3.4 therefore focus on social class as a structural location and as actively produced.

---

**Box 3.2**

---

'Men make their own history, but they do not make it as they please; they do not make it under self-selected circumstances, but under circumstances existing already, given and transmitted from the past.' (Marx, 1852: 329)

---

## 3.3 Socio-economic position as a structural location

The emphasis here is on socio-economic inequality as the product of social structures which exist outside and independent of people, bearing in on them as they make their way through their lives. Everyone is exposed to these structures; people can reduce, but not remove, their pervasive effects. Whether willingly or not, everyone is therefore socially positioned: everyone is slotted into a place in the social pecking order. Their place, in turn, allots them more or less of the resources – material and social – needed to do well and stay well in the societies of which they are part. This view of socio-economic inequality chimes with popular perceptions of British society. Surveys indicate that most people see Britain as a class-bound society, with its sharp inequalities working to the advantage of those privileged within it. Thus, around 60 per cent of adults in Britain believe that inequality persists because it benefits the rich and powerful. A majority, too, feel that Britain is too unequal: over 80 per cent regard the gap between those with high incomes and those with low incomes as too large (Bromley, 2003).

A perspective which emphasizes the societal origins of socio-economic inequality turns the spotlight on the social institutions which keep society going. In societies like the UK, these include legal systems regulating the ownership of property and the inheritance of wealth. They include, too, the education system, a labour market of powerful national and transnational corporations and the welfare state (Box 3.3). Many sociologists agree with Marx and point to the labour market as the major source and system of stratification. Social classes they argue 'are constituted not of people but of labour market situations . . . class is a characteristic not of people but of locations within the division of labour' (Harrison, 2006: 1).

Singly and together, these institutions both support and stratify people. On the one hand, these core institutions provide the resources which people need to survive and prosper. Children rely on the education system for the qualifications which are increasingly required to access well-paid jobs, the labour market is the primary source of income and the welfare state mediates access to services in 'cash and kind' in time of need and hardship.

---

**Box 3.3**

'The advanced capitalist societies are regulated by institutions that hardly existed in the era of industrialisation: the welfare state . . . mass education, and the modern corporation have emerged as important, if not decisive, institutional filters.' (Esping-Andersen, 1993: 8)

Such institutions therefore underwrite people's livelihoods. In Sen's terms, they influence people's capabilities: their freedom to do and achieve (see Chapter 1, section 1.3 for a discussion of Sen's capability perspective).

On the other hand, societal institutions provide resources in ways which allocate more to some than to others. In England, the majority of children are at school before the age of 5, beginning a long school career in which they can expect to take 70 external tests and examinations (Professional Association of Teachers, 2002). These tests and examinations rank children both in their own eyes and in the eyes of future employers (Reay, 2005). Similarly, the labour market requires intricate classificatory procedures to regulate appointment, advancement and job security, procedures which steer some workers towards well-paid and secure jobs – and restrict others to low-paid jobs punctuated by unemployment. A key function of the welfare state is to blunt the negative consequences of these labour market processes. But 'the welfare state is not just a mechanism that intervenes in, and possibly corrects, the structure of inequality; it is, in its own right, a system of stratification' (Esping-Andersen, 1990: 23). Its stratifying effects are most acutely felt by those who find themselves dependent on welfare services on an ongoing basis. Thus, studies charting the experience of claiming welfare benefits in the UK record how demeaning and energy-sapping the process of being endlessly categorized, re-assessed and monitored can be (Charlesworth, 2000). Expressed in Sen's terms, key societal institutions mediate people's freedoms to do and achieve; they facilitate opportunities for some groups to build lives that they value to a greater extent than for other groups.

So what is being suggested by those who regard socio-economic position as a structural location is that it is one produced, and held in place, by the stratifying processes of powerful institutions. In other words, institutions like the education system, the labour market and the broader structures of the welfare state 'sort people out'. In turn, these sorting institutions are regulated by government policies: on income and wealth, education and job creation, employment and social security. Policies are therefore a key lever for change: for moderating – or intensifying – inequalities which would otherwise result from unregulated labour markets and the inheritance of wealth. As subsequent chapters make clear, policies can and do make a difference to how unequal people's lives are.

## 3.4 Socio-economic position as actively produced

Sociologists have long recognized that social inequality is not simply 'out there', lurking in the social stratosphere and ensnaring hapless people who get caught in its nets. The processes which produce people's unequal positions – and thus the wider structure of socio-economic inequality – are also 'in here'.

Inequality is integrated into how we feel and how we act as we grow up and live our lives.

This does not mean that people talk about themselves in class terms. In the USA, for example, social class is absent from political discourse and popular understandings of how society works (Gimenez, 2006). Instead, ethnic and racial identities serves as oblique markers of social class: as Gans puts it, 'in a society that likes to see itself as classless, race comes in very handy as a substitute' (2005: 18). In the UK, most people recognize that they live in a class-based and class-bound society. But they still have difficulty in applying class labels to themselves. 'The absence of class as an articulated identity' (Bettie, 2000: 27) may reflect a widespread unease about defining oneself through the language of class (as upper class, middle class, or working class, for example). Studies report a reticence about owning up to one's privileged position and a parallel defensiveness about representing oneself as working class (Skeggs, 1997; Savage *et al.*, 2001). Additionally or alternatively, it may be because people are uncertain about what class labels are based on. While researchers tend to measure social class and socio-economic position along a single axis, like occupation, studies suggest that these concepts are popularly understood in more multidimensional terms. In one study, for example, participants used 14 criteria to define social class, including differences in wealth, education, occupation, housing and lifestyle as well as feelings of superiority and inferiority (Payne and Grew, 2005). This suggests that, while struggling to define it, people recognize that social class is threaded deeply into people's sense of who they are and where they belong.

Sociologists argue that people fashion these class identities and class positions as they go about their daily lives (Box 3.4). Through the rhythms and routines of everyday life – going to school, earning a living, caring for children – people 'reproduce the structure of which they are part, including its inequalities' (Blackburn and Prandy, 1997: 503). In this sense, everyone is

---

**Box 3.4**

'Inequality must be seen as embedded in a structure [that is] . . . reproduced through the circumstances and actions of those involved in it . . . The movement and action of individuals is the structure . . . Typically they will be socialised into the attitudes and behaviour appropriate to their position in their society, receive the appropriate form of education and training, move into typical early jobs, marry someone from a similar background, experience a typical career, in turn have children of their own and so on. All this happens by way of getting on with their lives, and as they do they reproduce the structure of which they are part, including its inequalities.' (Blackburn and Prandy, 1997: 502–3)

implicated in the processes which perpetuate inequality and thus are involved in sustaining their advantaged or disadvantaged position within it. But, as with so much else in life, not everyone enjoys the same opportunities to determine where they are going. Studies demonstrate that those born into privilege are more likely to experience themselves as agents of their own destiny; the sense of driving one's own life is harder to secure and to sustain for those struggling against disadvantage (Sennett and Cobb, 1973; Skeggs, 1997; Charlesworth, 2000).

Sociologists have drawn on the work of a French sociologist, Pierre Bourdieu, to illuminate the processes through which people produce the unequal positions in which they are located. Like other contemporary theorists, he argues that social class in post-industrial societies is forged not only through people's position in the labour market and their ownership of property. While economic power continues to be important, he suggests that class privilege also relies on other kinds of resources and, in particular, on the possession of cultural resources and command over social resources. He borrows the concept of capital from Marx to describe these different types of assets, extending it beyond the economic sphere to the cultural and social domain.

Bourdieu uses the concept of social capital to refer to social connections which enhance access to scarce resources, like good jobs and political influence. It therefore describes the networks secured by those on advantaged trajectories as they go through their lives – at school and university, at work and through marriage – which open doors to centres of power and influence.[1] His more influential concept of cultural capital is somewhat loosely defined. It includes the psychosocial resources which help people to succeed in the education system and in the labour market, and beyond these arenas, to assume positions of power in national politics and the global economy. Cultural capital is embodied in habitual ways of thinking, feeling and behaving, in what Bourdieu calls 'habitus'. The underlying idea is captured in Kate Fox's expose of social class in England (Box 3.5).

The habitual ways in which class distinction is lived and displayed do not remain constant: if lifestyles and consumption patterns are taken up more widely, they lose their prestige value. For example, in early twentieth-century Britain, it was those at the top of the class hierarchy who took up the new habit of cigarette smoking; they displayed their wealth, too, by not being engaged in physical labour (earning the label 'the leisured classes'). But as cigarette smoking and physical inactivity have become more widespread, class distinction has been increasingly expressed through not smoking and through taking exercise. Today, cigarette smoking and physical inactivity are markers of poverty rather than affluence (Sprotson and Primatesta, 2004).

Bourdieu developed the concepts of cultural capital and habitus to uncover the processes by which socio-economic inequality is maintained in post-industrial societies. These are societies whose wealth depends on the

---

**Box 3.5**

'We judge social class in much more subtle and complex ways . . . fine distinctions are applied to exactly what, where and how and with whom you eat and drink; the words you use and how you pronounce them; where and how you shop; the clothes you wear; the pets you keep; how you spend your free time; the chat up lines you use and so on . . . And one cannot talk at all without immediately revealing one's own social class . . . Your accent and terminology reveal the class you were born into and raised in, not anything you have achieved through your own talents or efforts. And whatever you do accomplish, your position on the class scale will always be identifiable by your speech, unless you painstakingly train yourself to use the pronunciation and vocabulary of a different class.' (Fox, 2004: 15, 73 and 82)

---

service sector, a sector which operates through relationships with clients, customers and consumers. In these people-oriented industries, sociological studies suggest that employers seek out and reward workers with particular kinds of social skills, leaving those without them struggling to find paid work. Thus, how a person looks, talks and behaves is seen to play an increasingly important part in the selection and promotion process, with employers looking beyond educational qualifications to 'such attributes as physical appearance, dress sense, accent, self-presentation, lifestyle and savoir faire, along with related "social" and "interpersonal" skills' (Erikson and Goldthorpe, 2002: 40). In Bourdieu's terms, what matters is cultural capital.

## 3.5 Childhood and parenting

Childhood is central to the accumulation and transmission of the capitals which matter in high-income societies – and thus to the broader social processes through which inequalities in socio-economic position are fashioned as people go about their lives. It is the time when cognitive skills (like thinking, learning and memory) are developed and when educational qualifications are secured. Bourdieu notes how habitus is laid down in childhood, with the body functioning as a 'living memory pad' (1990: 78).

The centrality of childhood to the persistence of class inequality has, inevitably, turned the spotlight on those most actively involved in child care and development. As Steadman observes, while a child's class position is conventionally defined by his or her father's occupation, it is women who materialize this position for their children and transmit it through their practices as mothers (Steadman, 1986: 55). Building on this insight, qualitative studies have described how the work that parents do to support their children's development is generative of social class.

Diane Reay's analyses have been a particularly important source of insight into this generative aspect of parenting (see, for example, Reay, 1998, 2004). Her ethnographic studies detail how mothers' class backgrounds influence their modes of engagement in their children's education. She suggests that middle-class mothers – those who have done well when they were at school and are bringing up their family on a secure income – have a confident and proactive approach, devoting time and money to helping their children at home and ensuring their learning needs are met at school. Thus one mother described 'the support I give him at home, hearing him read every night, doing homework with him, trying to get him the books he needs for his project' and noted that she had successfully secured 'extra support for him' at school (Reay, 2004: 78). Working-class mothers were much less likely to have the self-confidence to be actively engaged in their children's education at home or to negotiate individualized learning for their child at school. One mother expressed anxieties evident for many when she said 'I knew I should be playing a role in Darren's reading but I wasn't qualified. Therefore it put extra pressure on me because I was no good at reading myself, it was too important to handle and I'd get very upset and angry at Darren' (Reay 2004: 78). Another noted how her attempts to get extra help with reading for her son backfired: she was seen as demanding and her son consequently did not get the additional support she sought. As Reay concludes, both economic capital (money, homes with space and facilities for home-based learning) and cultural capital (self-assurance, particular kinds of linguistic and social skills) are needed to compensate for and modify state education, 'resources disproportionately located within middle class rather than working class families' (1998: 5).

Such detailed studies of the deployment of cultural capital provide an illustration of how advantage and disadvantage can be transmitted across generations. It highlights how different forms of capital are often mutually reinforcing. Parents with economic capital can invest in their children's education by providing facilities and materials to support learning at home (and beyond this, by living in areas with well regarded schools and by using private education). Their cultural capital can be deployed to maximize progress at school, thus further enhancing the rewards that their children secure from their economically privileged position. Not surprisingly, their children are well placed to gain educational qualifications and to acquire the types of cultural capital that employers are seen to increasingly value.

Ethnicity is deeply implicated in the process through which class advantage is maintained. Studies note that the cultural capital that white middle-class parents seek to protect and pass on to their children is specifically white and middle class, with parents using their economic resources and social networks to find schools that enrol enough children like their own (Byrne, 2006).

Community networks and a sense of cultural belonging can be equally, if not more, important for Caribbean and Asian children, and particularly for working-class children, as they negotiate their way through the education system (Reay, 2005; Reynolds, 2006). In the UK's Chinese community, parents, and the kinship network more broadly, have been found to generate cultural capital for their children by socializing them into a 'central narrative' of upward mobility (Archer and Francis, 2006). The expectation of children's upward mobility is instilled, in part, to compensate for the downward mobility that their parents endured when, as first-generation migrants, they were forced to take jobs below their levels of training and skills (Modood, 2004). The expectation is underwritten by supplementary schooling to enhance language skills and examination performance, and the result is levels of educational attainment which outstrip all other ethnic groups (DfES, 2003; Modood, 2004).

Of course, it is not only parents who are actively engaged in the reproduction of social class. Children and their teachers are also agents in the process. Here, studies have noted how young people without the kinds of cultural capital which are recognized and rewarded by the education system, struggle to remain confident and motivated. Long days, months, and years at school without the affirmation of teachers can fuel a powerful sense of exclusion, a sense which can dash ambitions and shape expectations for the future. In particular, it can encourage young people to self-select routes to adulthood which do not involve staying at school and taking examinations (see Chapters 8 and 9).

## 3.6 Conclusions

The chapter has examined the concept of socio-economic inequality, a concept more usually termed 'class inequality' in the disciplines which have made it a focus of study. It has noted that the economic and social changes which characterize today's rich societies led some social theorists to argue that social class has lost its grip on people's lives. However, the evidence points to persisting, rather than weakening, inequalities in people's opportunities to do well at school and in the labour market.

In explaining these persisting inequalities, social researchers have described how inequalities in socio-economic position are etched deeply into the social structure – and, at the same time, are produced by people going about their lives. Thus, on the one hand, studies have pointed to the role of social agencies and institutions, like the labour market and the education system, in the stratification process and the distribution of economic resources. On the other, studies have documented how socio-economic positions are individually and actively constructed, particularly through the parenting practices of mothers. Pierre Bourdieu's concept of 'cultural capital' (for example, in the form of social and linguistic skills and a strong sense of self-worth and entitlement) has proved particularly helpful here. Studies have highlighted how such capital can 'oil the wheels' of class advantage, enabling those who are well-off both to consolidate their privileges and to pass them on to their children. Conversely, restricted access to the kinds of cultural capital, which are recognized and rewarded at school and in the workplace, can leave children from poorer backgrounds multiply disadvantaged.

An appreciation that class inequality is produced and sustained by the interplay of social structure and individual agency is particularly important for understanding health inequalities. This is because people's bodies are sandwiched between the two. Class inequalities 'are manifest not simply in the form of differential access to economic, educational or cultural resources, but are embodied' (Shilling, 1993: 125). In consequence, 'class is always coded through bodily dispositions; the body is the most ubiquitous signifier of class' (Skeggs, 1997: 82). The chapter has pointed to some of the ways in which people embody their socio-economic position. It has noted that social class is embodied psychologically, through parents' sense of entitlement and self-efficacy in their interactions with the education system, and socially, in their self-presentation and 'people skills'. It is behaviourally embodied in child-care practices as well as in health behaviours like cigarette smoking. As signalled in Chapter 2, social class is also physically embodied: in trajectories of development through childhood and decline through adulthood, in health status and in patterns of disease and premature death. These multiple forms of embodiment are explored in later chapters of the book.

# 4  Measuring socio-economic position

## 4.1 Introduction

Chapter 3 discussed some key debates about socio-economic inequalities. These debates suggest that people's unequal socio-economic positions are both societally determined and individually generated: they are fashioned by individuals making their way in societies whose major institutions continuously stratify them. These unequal positions mean that people have unequal access to the resources which their societies value. In post-industrial societies like the UK, these resources are not confined to economic assets, like a well-paid job, financial investments and property. Various types of cultural capital also matter. This means that socio-economic position does not have a single determinant. Instead, it is constituted along a range of dimensions.

Socio-economic inequality can therefore be conceptualized as a multi-dimensional continuum. In broad terms, those with more of the resources which their society values – richer parents, more educational qualifications, higher-status jobs – will occupy positions towards the top end of the continuum, while those with less will be concentrated at its lower end. But it is very unlikely that two people will find themselves at identical points on the continuum, however similar their biographies. Nevertheless, they might expect to share some common ground: a similarity in their family backgrounds, for example, or educational histories or current jobs. It is this common ground which forms the basis of classifications of socio-economic position. The classifications group together broadly similar social backgrounds, educational profiles and occupations into socio-economic categories, which are then ranged along a continuum of differential social advantage (Blackburn and Prandy, 1997).

The chapter focuses on the classificatory process. It does so mindful of the fact that socio-economic inequality is part of a matrix of inequalities. Everyone also occupies unequal positions linked to their gender, cultural background and ethnic identity, sexuality and degree of impairment. Singly and together, these additional dimensions of inequality shape people's lives and their access to resources – and therefore their health. But the existence and influence of inequalities of gender, ethnicity, sexuality and disability have been eclipsed in social and health research. This is largely because the focus has been on those in the dominant positions of these unequal structures. Research, and the classificatory procedures on which it rests, has focused on white, straight and non-disabled men. While much of what is known about socio-economic and health inequalities derives from studies of this subgroup, they make up only a minority of the total population, at both national and global level.

Some UK examples may help to illustrate this partial perspective. The country is built out of ethnic diversity: it is a mix of people with different cultural heritages. Ethnicity, in turn, has multiple (and changing) dimensions, with religion and language often forming part of its fabric – as for instance in the meaning of being Welsh, Irish or Indian. The complexities of people's ethnic identities, however, have been largely invisible in the major sources of social and health data. It was not until the 1980s that a question on ethnic identity was included in major social and health surveys – and not until 1991 that a question was added to the UK Census. In response to the ethnicity question in the 2001 Census, around 8 per cent of the population and 12 per cent of young people did not classify themselves as white, a proportion which reached four in ten in London (APHO, 2005). But ethnicity is still not recorded on death certificates which, as Chapter 2 makes clear, underpin the most widely used measures of health. As a result, little is known about inequalities in life expectancy and premature mortality across ethnic groups or about socio-economic inequalities between and within ethnic groups for these basic measures of life and death.

Sexuality (or sexual orientation as it is called in official documents) provides another example. While around one in ten of the UK population report that they have had a sexual experience with a partner of the same sex (Erens *et al.*, 2003), information on how people understand and define their sexuality is not routinely collected. Questions about sexuality are still not included in the census, major surveys and data routinely gathered by welfare agencies. Further, until recently, a lesbian or gay couple were unable to record their cohabiting relationship in these key data sources. Cohabitation could only be heterosexual. As the major social survey, the *General Household Survey* put it, 'an informant can only be cohabiting with an unrelated member of the opposite sex' (OPCS, 1990: 262). In line with this assumption, gay men and lesbians who ticked the box marked 'living together as a couple' in the 1991 Census had their records changed at the data processing stage: 'cohabiting couples of the same sex were not recorded as such, instead, after clerical scrutiny of the forms, either the record of the sex of one of the couple or the relationship was changed' (Population Trends, 1993: 5). Today, however, same-sex cohabitation is increasingly recorded in social surveys, and the establishment of civil partnership in the UK is likely to encourage greater official recognition that not everyone is heterosexual.

As these examples suggest, dimensions other than socio-economic position have struggled to find a secure place in social research and official statistics. Against this background, sections 4.2 and 4.3 discuss the measurement and the measures of socio-economic position. It needs to be emphasized that the sections do not provide a comprehensive review. Their aim is to highlight some important measurement issues and introduce key measures used in the chapters which follow.

## 4.2 Measurement of socio-economic position

Information on socio-economic position is collected in the census and in social surveys using standardized questions which can be used to rank people according to (for example) their education, occupation or income. As this suggests, the measurement process treats socio-economic position as a property of the individual (as highest educational qualification, for instance, or current job) rather than – as sociologists have argued – a product of the societies in which they live. Similarly, 'tick box' questions represent gender and ethnicity as individual characteristics, not as dimensions of an unequal social structure. Cast in this way, it can be easy to mistake the individual level indicator for the societal-level concept: to lose sight of social position – of socio-economic, gender and ethnic positions, for example – as socially structured locations which unequally resource people's lives.

Epidemiologists, and health researchers more generally, have been criticized for this myopic view of social position. They are seen to individualize social position by detaching it from the structures of which it is part and reconfiguring it as an attribute of the individual (Krieger, 1994; Shim, 2000, 2002). This process means that socio-economic position – like ethnicity or gender – disappears as a manifestation of the social structure and re-emerges as an individual risk factor for disease. As Janet Shim puts it, 'epidemiology thereby renders invisible the very social relations of power structuring material and psychic conditions and life chances that contribute to the stratification of health and illness' (2002: 134).

It is not only the process of measurement which has been criticized. Concerns have also been raised about the measures themselves. The standard classificatory schema has been designed by state officials who occupy the privileged categories in the classificatory systems that they develop. The tacit reference group is therefore white, heterosexual and non-disabled men in higher professional and managerial jobs. As Chapter 2, section 2.3 noted, measures of disability have been criticized for blurring the distinction between

functional impairments and socially imposed barriers, a distinction fundamental to the experience and politics of disability. Ethnicity – a multifaceted
category in which a sense of shared history, language and religion can all play
a part – is reduced to a classification which has 'white' as its implicit reference
group. Ethnicity is therefore assigned to those who fall outside it (as in 'minority ethnic group') (Frankenburg, 1997). Thus, the 2001 Census asked 'what is
your ethnic group?' through a checklist headed by 'white' and with non-white
categories listed beneath it (for example, 'Asian or Asian British' and 'Black or
Black British Caribbean'). As Hickman notes, 'by definition, ethnic minorities
are British subjects but their classification as members of minorities securely
locates them in a subordinate position in the hierarchy of "Britishness" '
(2005: 22). In consequence, and not surprisingly, people's identities are often
in deep conflict with official definitions of who they are (Steadman, 1986).
The sense of disjuncture is most acutely felt by those allocated to subordinate categories, for example, by those allocated to 'unskilled' occupational
categories and to 'lower' socio-economic groups, (Skeggs, 1997), those defined
as disabled (Oliver, 1996) or as 'not white' (Frankenburg, 1997).

One consequence of designing classifications with a particular subgroup
in mind is that they can work less well for other groups. For example, the
associations between measures of socio-economic position, like education,
occupation and income, evident for white non-disabled men may not hold
true for other groups. It cannot therefore be assumed that a given level of
educational attainment (a degree, for example) will secure an equivalent level
of occupation and income for everyone. There is, in the language of social
research, a 'non-equivalence' of socio-economic measures. Box 4.1 gives some
examples. As it notes, the employment and income gains for a given level of
education are typically lower for women than men, for some minority ethnic
groups than for the white majority, and for people with impairments when
compared with the rest of the population (see Box 4.1). Underlying this non-
equivalence is social inequality: those in advantaged positions derive a higher
return on education and occupation than those in subordinate positions.

---

**Box 4.1**

- a given level of education is associated with lower rates of employment for
  women than for men (Berthoud and Blekesaune, 2006)
- a Bangladeshi with a degree is estimated to have the same risk of poverty as
  a white person with no qualifications (Berthoud, 1998)
- among those in paid work and with the same level of educational qualifications, a disabled person is more likely to be low paid than one who is non-
  disabled (Burchardt, 2005).

## 4.3 Measures of socio-economic position

Information relating to individuals, their households and the areas in which they live are all used to measure people's socio-economic position. Individual and household indicators are typically referred to as measures of socio-economic position (or social class or socio-economic status). For area-level measures, these terms are less often used, with terms like 'living standards' and 'area deprivation' preferred instead.

### Occupation

In the UK, occupation has long been used to allocate people to socio-economic groups. The rationale is that paid work is the most important determinant of 'the life-fates of the majority of individuals and their families in advanced industrial societies' (Crompton, 1993: 120). This makes current occupation a 'reasonable indicator of social position' (see Box 4.2).

Occupation is used to measure the socio-economic position not only of the individual worker but of other household members as well. The traditional way of deriving this collective class position has been through the occupation of 'the man of the house'. In the surveys and censuses which marked the development of social research in Britain, women and children were ascribed the social class of the men they lived with. It is an approach which, as critics have noted, erases inequalities between members of the household – in access to education, in the division of paid and unpaid work as well as in the distribution of income. In so doing, it masks the gender divisions on which family life is built and through which the occupation of 'the man of the house' becomes the primary marker of the class position of his female partner and their children. Partly in response to these criticisms, alternative ways of deriving household social class have been developed. One approach identifies a 'household reference person' whose occupation is likely to have the greatest impact on living standards and consumption patterns of household members (Rose and Pevalin, 2003). To identify the dominant occupation, the partner with a

---

**Box 4.2**

'Occupation (usually combined with employment status) is a reasonable indicator of overall social position. This is because the life chances of individuals and families depend mainly on their position in the social division of labour and on the material and symbolic advantages they derive from it.' (Rose and Pevalin, 2003: 17)

current full-time job is selected in preference to one who is economically inactive or in part-time work; if both partners are in full-time employment, household social class is determined by the occupation of the partner in the higher status job. Since men typically score higher on these criteria than women, women living with men again typically find themselves assigned a socio-economic position on the basis on their partner's occupation (Crompton, 1993).

An alternative is to take the individual, rather than the household, as the unit of measurement. However, this is not without problems. While most adults have a current or previous job, it leaves children and young people who have yet to enter the labour market outside the classificatory schema – and thus outside the class structure. Those with intermittent and interrupted work histories also find themselves ambiguously located, an ambiguous location shared by many women, unemployed people and people with long-term impairments. Together, these groups make up the majority of the population.

Whether occupations are treated as a property of individuals or are used to measure the socio-economic position of the household as whole, classifications need to be devised to group and categorize occupations. An early schema divided the British population into 'three great classes of inhabitants': 'the gentry and professional people and their families', 'farmers, tradesmen and their families' and 'artisans, labourers and their families'. The class gradients in health which the schema revealed are discussed in Chapter 5 (see Figure 5.6). These three great classes were extended and formalized in 'the classification of occupations' developed by the Registrar General and introduced into the 1911 Census. This grouped occupations considered to require similar levels of skill. The occupational classes ranged from social class 1 (labelled 'upper and middle class' in the 1911 social class classification) to social class V ('unskilled manual'), with additional classes added for textile workers, miners and agricultural workers (Registrar General, 1913). By the early 1920s, the classification had evolved into a simpler fivefold division of occupational classes and became the dominant measure of socio-economic position in the UK (Table 4.1). For instance, it was used in Table 2.2 (class inequalities in infant mortality) and Figure 2.3 (class inequalities in deaths from heart disease) – and features prominently in the chapters which follow.

In 2001, a new system for measuring socio-economic position was launched. The National Statistics-Socio-Economic Classification (NS-SEC) replaced the Registrar General's social classes as the UK's official classification. It places occupations into groups (called 'operational categories') on the basis of their dominant employment relations and conditions, such as whether wages or salaries are paid, how much job security and autonomy workers have, and whether there is a career structure and prospects for promotion (Rose and Pevalin, 2003). Table 4.2 describes the simplified typologies which can be derived from the classification. The main NS-SEC schema has eight

**Table 4.1** Registrar General's social class classification

| Social class | Examples of occupations |
| --- | --- |
| I Professional occupations | Doctor, accountant |
| II Managerial and intermediate occupations | Teacher, manager |
| III Skilled occupations | |
| NM: non-manual | Secretary, sales representative |
| M: manual | Bus driver, electrician |
| IV Partly-skilled occupations | Security guard, assembly worker |
| V Unskilled occupations | Office cleaner, labourer |

**Table 4.2** National Statistics-Socio-Economic Classification (NS-SEC): nine-, five-and three-class versions

| Nine classes | Five classes | Three classes |
| --- | --- | --- |
| 1.1 Large employers and higher managerial occupations | | |
| 1.2 Higher professional occupations | | |
| | 1 Managerial and professional occupations | 1 Managerial and professional occupations |
| 2 Lower managerial and professional occupations | | |
| 3 Intermediate occupations | 2 Intermediate occupations | |
| | | 2 Intermediate occupations |
| 4 Small employers and own account workers | 3 Small employers and own account workers | |
| | 4 Lower supervisory and technical occupations | |
| 5 Lower supervisory and technical occupations | | |
| | | 3 Routine and manual occupations |
| 6 Semi-routine occupations | 5 Semi-routine and routine occupations | |
| 7 Routine occupations | | |
| 8 Never worked and long-term unemployed | Never worked and long-term unemployed | Never worked and long-term unemployed |

*Source:* Rose and Pevalin, 2003. Reprinted by permission of Sage Publilcations Ltd from Rose and Pevalin's *A Researcher's Guide to the National Statistics Socio-Economic Classification* (© Sage Publications 2003)

socio-economic classes, which can be collapsed into a five-class schema. In contrast to earlier measurement scales, both of these break with the assumption that social class and socio-economic position are hierarchically ordered categories. But as Table 4.2 indicates, the NS-SEC's socio-economic classes can be simplified into a three-category measure: managerial and professional, intermediate, and routine and manual. While those designing the new classification do not recommend it, the three-class schema can be treated as hierarchical.

## Education

Education is the principal measure of socio-economic position in Europe and the USA, and one with a number of advantages. In rich societies with universal education systems, it provides an inclusive measure for the adult population. This means that most adults can be classified by years of, and age of, leaving full-time education as well as by highest educational qualification. With most people completing their education by their early twenties, education is also a stable measure of position. In contrast to occupation or income, it changes little across adulthood. Finally, because it is typically set by early adulthood, educational level provides a measure of socio-economic position which is independent of subsequent health status. In other words, an individual's educational level does not change if they go on to develop a chronic illness which forces them into a lower status job or out of the labour market. This is particularly important for studies seeking to establish the contribution of socio-economic disadvantage to future health.

However, education-based measures are not without their drawbacks. First, years and levels of education have a somewhat ambiguous status as measures of adult position. This is because, strictly speaking, education anticipates, rather than represents, adult socio-economic position: it lies on the pathway linking parental social class (class of origin) and own social class (class of destination). As Chapter 3, section 3.4 signalled and Chapter 8, section 8.4 makes clear, a child's educational trajectory is powerfully shaped by the socio-economic circumstances of their family – and powerfully shapes their future position in the labour market. Social and health researchers have therefore treated education as both a proxy for childhood circumstances and a marker of adult socio-economic position.

Second, because governments set the age of leaving full-time education and determine the structure of qualifications, changes in educational policy can produce marked changes in the socio-economic profile of the population. For example, in Britain in the 1940s, 90 per cent of women fell into the lowest educational category, with no secondary education and no educational qualifications (Douglas and Blomfield, 1958). Among young women at school today, full-time secondary education is compulsory to the age of 16 and a

third can expect to secure the qualifications they need to enter higher education (Machin, 2003). While useful for cross-sectional studies, educational
measures need to be used with caution in analyses of inequalities over time
(see Chapter 8).

Third, for some groups there is likely to be little variation in educational
levels. For example, adults with intellectual disabilities are heavily concentrated in the 'no qualifications' category. As a result, education-based measures
have limited capacity to detect differences in their socio-economic circumstances – and thus limited capacity to measure health inequalities in these
groups (Emerson *et al.*, 2006).

### Household income

People's incomes – from earnings, occupational pensions, savings and investments as well as from welfare benefits – are the major determinant of their
living standards. These incomes are usually measured at household level,
with household income providing both a marker of socio-economic position
and the data through which poverty is measured. Household income can be
measured in various ways. Market income is income before direct taxes have
been subtracted and state transfers, like welfare benefits, have been added.
Disposable income is income after account is taken of taxes and transfers,
and therefore more accurately describes the income that households have
available to spend. Housing costs, like rent and mortgage repayments are often
deducted from this standard measure of income ('income after housing costs').
Housing costs vary widely across regions, eating more deeply into disposable
income in some regions (south-east England, for example) than in others (the
ex-industrial regions of northern England and south Wales). In addition,
because different types of household need different levels of income to achieve
the same standard of living, incomes are adjusted ('equivalized') to take account
of the size and composition of the household. However, no adjustment is
made for additional costs resulting from long-term illness and impairment.

Income data can be used to divide the population into income deciles
(tenths), quintiles (fifths) and tertiles (thirds), an approach widely used in
studies of health inequalities (see Chapter 6). Household income can be used,
too, to set a poverty line. The poverty line can be defined either in terms of
the minimum incomes people need in order to survive or in the context of
the incomes of the population as a whole. The former approach rests on an
absolute concept, and the latter on a relative concept, of poverty.

The USA is one of the few high-income societies where the official poverty
line is an absolute one. The poverty threshold is based on the minimum estimated cost of a basket of basic items (Fisher, 1992) and represents an income
well below that judged both by researchers and by the general public as neces-
sary to 'live decently' and to avoid hardship (Magnuson and Duncan, 2002:

96). This threshold is uprated in line with inflation but, as an absolute poverty line, not with average incomes. As the USA has got richer, the poverty line has therefore fallen relative to average income, with the living standards of those officially defined as poor slipping further behind the rest of the population. With poverty thresholds failing to keep step with rising incomes among middle- and higher-income families, individuals and families living below it are becoming increasingly economically isolated (Mishel *et al.*, 2006).

In Europe, poverty lines are usually defined relative to the incomes of the population as a whole. The European Union (EU) has adopted such a relative concept of poverty, with each member state having a national poverty line based on its average household income. There are two major ways in which average household income is measured. *Mean income* is calculated by dividing the income of all the households in the population by the total number of households. Poverty lines based on mean income are typically set at an income below half (50 per cent) of mean household income. *Median income* is the income of the household at the mid-point of the income distribution: if all the households are ranged from poorest to richest, the median income is that of the household in the middle. Poverty lines are often drawn at either 50 per cent or 60 per cent of national median income: adults and children living in households with incomes below the threshold are defined as poor.

The distinction between mean and median income is important in societies where the income distribution is skewed, with a small proportion of super-rich households raising national mean income well above national median income. This has long been the case in Britain. In 2005, mean income stood at £427 a week, 1.2 times higher than the median income of £349. Because of the gap between the two measures, two-thirds of the population live in households below the national average as measured by mean income. Partly for this reason, the government has shifted from mean income to median income as the basis of its poverty line, with households below 60 per cent of median household income defined as poor. Table 4.3 gives examples of this poverty line in 2004–5 for different household types, both before and after the deduction of housing costs. Measured after housing costs, 20 per cent of the British population, and 27 per cent of children, were living in poverty in 2005 (Brewer *et al.*, 2006).

Information on household income is not only used to measure how many households fall below particular income thresholds. It is also used to indicate how equally a country's income is distributed between households. One popular measure of the income distribution is the Gini coefficient, developed by Corrado Gini, an Italian statistician. It measures the degree of equality on a scale from 0 to 100 (or 0 to 1). A value of 0 indicates complete income equality: after adjustment for household size and composition, everyone has the same household income. If the Gini coefficient was 100, one household would have all the income. Differences in the methods used to measure income – using

**Table 4.3** Poverty line of 60 per cent median income for different households before and after housing costs, Britain, 2004–5

|  | Weekly income before housing costs | Weekly income after housing costs |
|---|---|---|
| Single person | £128 | £100 |
| Couple with no children | £210 | £183 |
| Lone parent with one child aged 8 | £176 | £142 |
| Lone parent with two children aged 1 and 3 | £184 | £146 |
| Couple with one child aged 8 | £258 | £225 |
| Couple with two children aged 1 and 3 | £266 | £228 |

*Source:* Brewer *et al.*, 2006. Reproduced under the terms of the click-use licence

**Table 4.4** Gini coefficient (GDP per capita, PPP US$) for selected countries 1999–2001

| | |
|---|---|
| Sweden | 25.0 |
| Norway | 25.8 |
| Canada | 33.1 |
| Sri Lanka | 33.2 |
| UK | 36.0 |
| United States | 40.8 |
| Ghana | 40.8 |
| Nicaragua | 43.1 |
| China | 44.7 |
| South Africa | 57.8 |

*Source:* UNDP, 2005, table 15. Permission applied for

market rather than disposable income or not adjusting for differences in household composition, for example – means that caution needs to be exercised when comparing the Gini coefficients derived from different studies.

With this cautionary note in mind, Table 4.4 describes broad patterns of income inequality between countries. The data are based on per capita gross domestic product (GDP), expressed in US$ and adjusted to achieve purchasing power parity (PPP) by taking account of price differences between countries. As a general pattern, poorer countries have greater income inequalities than richer ones. Thus, as Table 4.4 suggests, the Gini coefficients for countries in Europe tend to be lower than in Africa, Asia and South America (Birdsall, 2006; Sáinz, 2006). But as the table indicates, there are poor countries with low Gini coefficients, and rich countries with levels of income inequality comparable to those found in much poorer countries. Across these national differences, however, is a global trend to greater income inequality within countries. The trend is evident in many high-income countries, including the USA and the UK, in high-growth low- and middle-income countries like India and China, and particularly in the post-Communist economies of the former Soviet Union and Eastern Europe (Birdsall, 2006). In the USA and the UK, the Gini coefficient surged upwards from the late 1970s and continued to climb through the 1980s and 1990s. In both countries, it remains at historically high levels (Brewer *et al.*, 2006; Mishel *et al.*, 2006).

### Area-based measures

Rich people tend to live in areas which have a higher proportion of rich people, while poorer people are over represented in places where their neighbours are also poor. These residential concentrations mean that people's socio-economic circumstances can be measured using indicators of the areas in which they live. The spatial unit can range from a small area, like a neighbourhood, through larger units, like countries, to global regions.

At the local and sub-national level, indicators are often constructed from a range of markers of disadvantage. One example is the *Indices of Multiple Deprivation* used in the UK which combine indicators across a range of domains – including income, employment, housing and health – into a single deprivation score (ODPM, 2004). At the level of countries and global regions, single measures of people's living conditions are more widely used. Gross domestic product and gross national income (GNI)[1] per capita are examples. Gross domestic product measures the value of goods and services produced within a country, whether by its residents or by firms based there; GNI measures the value of goods and services produced by the country's citizens, whether they are living inside or outside of the country. Average income per person is calculated by dividing these measures by the population denominator and adjusted for price differences between countries to achieve 'purchasing power parity'. Typically, per capita incomes are expressed in US dollars.

Gross national income per capita has been used to classify a country's economy as 'high income' 'middle income' or 'low income'. The categories are based on the World Bank's lending criteria, with the thresholds updated annually in line with estimates of international inflation (World Bank, 2006). Examples of countries in these broad income groups are given in Table 4.5. Around 60 per cent of the world's population live in low-income countries, where GNI per capita is equivalent to $875 a year or less (2005 thresholds). Around a quarter live in middle-income countries, with average incomes between $875 and $10,725. Less than one-sixth of the global population lives in high-income countries, like those in North America and western Europe, where GNI per person is $10,725 or more (World Bank DEP, 2006). Countries

**Table 4.5** High-, middle- and low-income countries in 2006: some examples

| High income | Middle income | Low income |
|---|---|---|
| Australia | Brazil | Bangladesh |
| Greece | China | Ghana |
| Japan | Jamaica | India |
| Netherlands | Nicaragua | Nigeria |
| Sweden | South Africa | Sudan |
| United States | Ukraine | Vietnam |

*Source:* adapted from World Bank website, 2006

like the UK and the USA are at the top end of the high-income range, with per capita incomes many times higher than the income threshold.

The World Bank has also established an international poverty line. This is based on the typical poverty line in low-income countries in the mid-1980s, updated in 1993 and adjusted to take account of inflation. People living on less than $1 a day (updated in 1993 to $1.08) are defined as living in 'extreme poverty'; those living on less than $2 a day are defined as poor. The measure is not without its weaknesses (see Reddy and Pogge, 2005, for a review). But it underlines the scale of global income inequality. On this measure, 23 per cent of the population of low- and middle-income countries are in extreme poverty; when less than $2 a day is taken as the poverty line, the proportion rises to 56 per cent (World Bank, 2003). The Human Development Index (HDI) has been developed as 'a powerful alternative to income as a summary measure of human wellbeing' (UNDP, 2005: 214). Underpinned by Sen's capability perspective, it is designed to measure the quality of people's lives along 'three basic dimensions of human development': a long and healthy life, as measured by life expectancy at birth; knowledge, as measured by the adult literacy rate and the combined gross enrolment ratio for primary, secondary and tertiary schools; and a decent standard of living, as measured by GDP per capita (UNDP, 2005: 214).

Area-based measures of people's circumstances are often the only measures available, and are therefore widely used in both national and international studies of health inequalities. However, they are not without their drawbacks. First, areas are socially mixed. Within poor areas there are many richer people, while rich areas are home to many poorer people. Analyses of poor children in the USA suggest that only one in six live in high-poverty urban neighbourhoods, defined as neighbourhoods where 40 per cent or more of residents live in households below the poverty line (Magnuson and Duncan, 2002: 98). Further, the overlap between household-level and area-level poverty is not consistent across ethnic groups. In the UK, levels of residential concentration are lower among white groups than among Caribbeans and

Indians, and are at their highest among Pakistanis (Robinson and Reeve, 2006).

Second, people's perceptions of their neighbourhood do not necessarily match the official ratings. African-Caribbeans and south Asians are more likely than whites to live in inner-city areas with high scores on the official deprivation indices. But those living in these areas are more likely to rate the availability of neighbourhood amenities and services highly than are white groups in more affluent areas (Bajekal *et al.*, 2004). In line with other studies, this suggests that residential concentration ('group density') may bring important material and social benefits for minority ethnic groups (Reynolds, 2006). Conversely, the health benefits of living in a better-off but largely white area may be wiped out by the loss of a protective and supportive community in which one feels accepted and valued (Mullings and Wali, 2001).

Third, because people move in and out of areas, comparisons of areas over time will be based on changing rather than stable populations. Taking account of inward and outward migration in analyses of health inequalities is complicated by the fact that these patterns of migration are not random. As a general rule, people who leave poor areas have better health than those who stay, and those moving out of affluent areas tend to be in poorer health than those they leave behind. This process of selective migration contributes to the spatial concentration of social deprivation and poor health (Brimblecombe *et al.*, 2000; Norman *et al.*, 2005).

Finally, area-based measures of people's socio-economic position mean that health influences operating at the individual and household level cannot be separated from those operating at the area level. The evidence suggests that individual and household circumstances are the more powerful predictors of health, but that areas have a small additional effect (Leventhal and Brooks-Gunn, 2000; Pickett and Pearl, 2001). This suggests that measures of individual and household circumstances are to be preferred in studies concerned with mapping and understanding their health effects.

## 4.4 Conclusions

This chapter has explored some of the issues which influence the measurement and measures of socio-economic position. It is an exploration which suggests that the task of finding appropriate indicators is complex and, as yet, unfinished. Social and health researchers work with a range of imperfect measures, trying to remain alert to their limitations while seeking to exploit their strengths.

What the review of measures makes clear is that socio-economic inequality is only partly captured by the indicators used to measure it. Further, the indicators tend to work better for some groups than others. For example, they capture the nature and scale of socio-economic inequalities among white men with greater precision than among white women and non-white groups. But for all groups, socio-economic indicators serve as markers for a concept which they partially, but never wholly, represent. Thus, a strong association between an indicator like educational qualifications and health does not mean that having a degree keeps one healthy while having no qualifications causes disease. Similarly, a strong association between the occupation of the father and the health of their children does not demonstrate that parental working conditions directly cause childhood injuries and illnesses. In these two examples, strong associations signal only that social factors which vary in line with educational qualifications and father's occupation may damage health and influence children's exposure to environmental danger and disease. These underlying social factors may not only be unmeasured; they may also be, as yet, unknown. Nonetheless, they hold the key to understanding why low educational qualifications is predictive of heart disease and father's occupation is linked to deaths in childhood.

Mindful of the gaps in measurement and understanding, Part 2 of the book investigates the strong associations between the measures of socio-economic position and health discussed in this chapter and Chapter 2. It looks at health inequalities between and within countries as well as over time and across changes in patterns of disease. Focusing on high-income countries, Part 3 presents evidence which sheds light on the causes of socio-economic inequalities in people's circumstances and in their health.

# PART 2
## Patterns

Part 2 sets people's unequal health in a geographical and historical perspective. Chapter 5 reviews evidence of inequalities in survival between countries, within countries and over time, with the UK taken as the focus of the historical review. Chapter 6 describes the unequal patterning of health across changes in the patterns of disease, both within high-income countries and in a global context.

# 5   Health inequalities: global, national and historical

## 5.1 Introduction

There is a wealth of evidence on how people's health is patterned by their social circumstances. But the evidence base is heavily tilted towards richer countries in which only a minority of the world's population live. In part, this is because these countries have more comprehensive data collection systems. In England and Wales, national registration systems for births and deaths have been in place since 1837. One hundred and seventy years on, the functioning vital registration systems required to measure life expectancy are estimated to cover only one in three deaths worldwide (Lopez *et al.*, 2001). However, the expansion of data collection systems for child health means that considerably more is known about the health of children than the health of adults in low- and middle-income countries. In consequence, death rates among children under the age of 5 are widely regarded as more reliable than other measures of population health (Lopez *et al.*, 2001).

However, the lack of evidence on health inequalities in poorer countries cannot be wholly explained by the limitations of their national data collection systems. It is also due to the targeting of research funding at the world's richest and healthiest populations. It has been estimated that, of the total volume of global health research funded by the public and private sector, less than 10 per cent is devoted to improving the health of 90 per cent of the world's population. This has been termed the '90/10' gap (Commission on Health Research for Development, 1990). But global health inequalities are so stark that even the paucity of data cannot disguise them. The first section of the chapter describes these stark inequalities.

The chapter then highlights health inequalities within countries before taking an historical perspective on people's unequal health. Evidence of a link between poor conditions and poor health dates back to ancient China, Greece and Egypt (Krieger 1997; Whitehead, 1997). But data have only been systematically collected since the mid-nineteenth century, and predominantly in the early-industrializing nations of northern Europe and North America. Britain, the first industrializing nation, has comparatively good historical records. While not necessarily representative of patterns elsewhere, it provides an insight into how inequalities persist over time and despite improvements in health in all socio-economic groups.

The indicators of socio-economic circumstances used in these sections were outlined in Chapter 4, section 4.3. They include measures of average living standards, like gross domestic product (GDP) and gross national income (GNI) per capita. The latter is used to define countries as high income, middle income or low income (World Bank, 2006). Within-country indicators include education, occupation and household income. The measures of health discussed in the sections below were outlined in Chapter 2, sections 2.2 and 2.3, and include life expectancy at birth, death rates among children under the age of 5 and self-assessed health.

## 5.2 Global health inequalities

Global life expectancy is at its highest recorded level. In 2001, it reached 66.7 years, an increase of eight years in two decades (UNDP, 2003). In the early decades of the twentieth century, life expectancy increased most rapidly in high-income countries in the face of a rapid decline in communicable diseases. From the middle decades, the most rapid improvements in life expectancy occurred in regions below the global average: in Africa, Latin America and the Caribbean and, particularly, Asia. As Figure 5.1 indicates, the result was

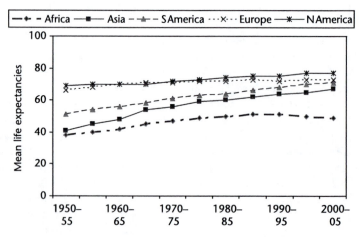

**Figure 5.1**  Mean life expectancies in different world regions 1950–2005

*Source:* Dorling *et al.*, 2006, table 1

a narrowing of global health inequalities between northern industrialized and southern agrarian countries between the 1950s and the 1980s (Labonte and Schrecker, 2005; Dorling *et al.*, 2006).

However from the 1980s, this global convergence in health faltered and a different pattern began to emerge. Life expectancy in Asia, the Middle East and north Africa has continued to rise, with levels of health moving closer to those in the high-income countries of Europe and North America. However in sub-Saharan Africa, the steady increase in life expectancy stalled at a point where life expectancy was still under 50 years. It is a region of the world in which the HIV/AIDS epidemic is dragging down life expectancy. In South Africa, for example, life expectancy stood at 47 years in 2001; 20 years earlier, it had been 57 (World Bank, 2003). It is a region, too, which is estimated to spend two to four times as much each year on servicing debts as on providing its population with education and health care (Labonte and Schrecker, 2006: 15).

Behind these global trends and regional histories lies a deeper relationship between national wealth and population health (Box 5.1). It is relationship captured in Table 5.1. The table charts the patterns of life expectancy and the proportion of children dying before their fifth birthday in low-income, middle-income and high-income countries. As it indicates, there is a 20-year difference in life expectancy between low-income countries (59 years) and high-income countries (78 years). Similarly, death rates among children in the world's poorest countries dwarf those in middle-income and high-income

---

**Box 5.1**

'Global inequality takes many dimensions. Not only is there great inequality across the peoples of the world in material standards of living, but there are also dramatic inequalities in health. The inhabitants of poorer countries not only have lower real incomes, but they are also more often sick, and they live shorter lives.' (Deaton, 2006: 1)

---

**Table 5.1**  Life expectancy at birth and under-5 mortality in low-income, middle-income and high-income countries, 2001

|  | *Life expectancy at birth* | *Under-5 mortality (deaths per 1000)* |
| --- | --- | --- |
| Low income | 59 | 121 |
| Middle income | 70 | 38 |
| High income | 78 | 7 |

*Source:* adapted from World Bank, 2003, table 2.20

countries. In low-income countries, one child in eight does not live to their fifth birthday; in high-income countries, one child in 143 dies before the age of 5 (World Bank, 2003). Shorter lives are often spent in poor health and with disabilities (see Chapter 2, section 2.3 for a discussion of impairment and disability). In sub-Saharan Africa, the region of the world with the lowest life expectancy, it is estimated that 18 per cent of the average life span is spent living with disabilities; in countries where life expectancy is high, like Japan, the proportion is around 8 per cent (Mathers *et al.*, 2000).

Table 5.1 points to a strong relationship between a nation's wealth and the health of its people. This relationship was highlighted by Samuel Preston in an analysis of the association between GDP per person and life expectancy published 30 years ago (Preston, 1975). The contemporary patterns of national wealth and population health are captured in Figure 5.2. It gives examples of countries lying along the 'Preston curve', with the examples drawn from low-income countries (Tanzania, Ghana), middle-income countries (Brazil) and high-income countries (Sweden). As Figure 5.2 indicates, when GDP is low, increases are strongly associated with improvements in life expectancy: at this point in the income distribution, the line linking income and health is almost vertical. Among richer countries, the curve flattens out, with higher incomes bringing diminishing health benefits. As this suggests, the marginal health gains of extra income are far greater at the lower end of the income range. It is a conclusion which lends support to the view that 'redistribution of income

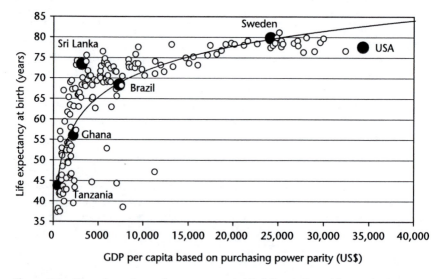

**Figure 5.2** Gross domestic product per person in US dollars (adjusted for purchasing power parity) and life expectancy in 159 countries, 2001

*Source:* World Bank, 2003

towards the poor will improve their average health by more than the loss of health among the rich' (Deaton, 2003: 115).

While national wealth and population health are strongly linked, they are not perfectly correlated. Figure 5.2 includes 'outlier' countries with lower or higher life expectancies than their wealth would predict. An example of a country where levels of health do not match its levels of wealth is the USA. In the early 2000s, the world's richest country had a lower life expectancy (77.0 years) than countries with much lower GDP, like Sweden (79.7 years) and Japan (80.7 years), and an infant mortality rate which was more than twice as high as these countries (World Bank, 2003). Among the complex of factors explaining the USA's poorer health record is an economic system built on minimal state intervention in the labour market and in welfare provision. With respect to labour market intervention, institutions to support collective bargaining and to protect wages and working conditions are relatively under-developed (Smeeding, 2002). With respect to welfare provision, the USA devotes a smaller proportion of its GDP than other high-income countries to supporting those unable to earn their way out of poverty, either in the form of cash benefits or services (OECD, 2005). Under-investment in employment protection and welfare provision combine to keep poverty rates (as measured by 50 per cent of median income) and income inequality appreciably higher than in other rich countries (UNDP, 2005; see also Table 4.4). High rates of poverty and marked income inequalities, in turn, exert a downward drag on life expectancy: as Deaton observes, 'if a rich country has a lot of poor people, it will have lower average health relative to its per capita income' (Deaton, 2003: 118).

An example of a country which combines low GDP with high life expectancy is Sri Lanka. As Figure 5.2 indicates, Sri Lanka's GDP is half that of Brazil, but it has a higher life expectancy (73.1 years compared to 68.1 years in Brazil). Sri Lanka also has a lower infant mortality rate (17 vs 31 per 1000) and a lower rate of under-5 mortality (15 vs 35 per 1000) (UNDP, 2003; World Bank, 2003). The key to its success has been identified as its equity-oriented approach to economic and social development (Fernando, 2000; Mills *et al.*, 2001). Thus, in contrast to the USA, Sri Lanka has linked economic growth to income redistribution by devoting a relatively high proportion of its national wealth to poverty alleviation (Mills *et al.*, 2001; WHO, 2004). As a result, the level of income inequality is low compared to low- and middle-income countries; it also compares well to levels in high-income countries (see Table 4.4). Sri Lanka invested, too, in primary education and public health provision from the early decades of the twentieth century, and the universal provision of free or heavily subsidized rice was introduced in the early 1940s (Drèze and Sen, 1989). The result is a country which has secured population-wide access to key health resources. Thus, literacy rates are high (90 per cent) and over 75 per cent of the population have access to safe drinking water. In addition, nearly 100 per cent of pregnant women receive antenatal care and are attended at birth by trained personnel, and over 80 per cent of children receive the full complement of immunizations by their first birthday (World Bank, 2003; WHO, 2004; UNDP, 2005). Rates of infectious disease, including HIV/AIDS, are also low (World Bank, 2003; WHO, 2004).

Kerala is often cited as a sub-national example of the extent to which policies matter (Sen, 1999). Thankappan (2001) provides an instructive analysis of this Indian state, which, with a per capita income around 1 per cent that of the richest countries, has achieved high standards of population health. For example in 2000, life expectancy stood at 76 years for women and 70 years for men: in the USA, life expectancy was 80 and 74 years, respectively. As in Sri Lanka, Kerala's health achievements are attributed to the combination of its relatively equitable distribution of wealth and economic resources, on the one hand, and its high levels of state investment in education and health, on the other (Thankappan, 2001). Examples include land reforms distributing land to the poorest and a system for distributing food at subsidized prices. At the same time, publicly funded services have been expanded to support women's education (female literacy rates of 87 per cent) and access to health care (97 per cent institutional deliveries) (Thankappan and Valiathan, 1998; Thankappan, 2001).

As the examples of the USA, Sri Lanka and Kerala suggest, the relationship between national wealth and population health is not a direct and simple one. Rather, the relationship appears to be mediated by government policies. In the USA, for example, redistributive institutions have not been developed on the scale found in European countries (Taylor-Gooby, 2005). It therefore lacks the institutional capacity to harness national wealth and direct it towards welfare interventions which level up living standards. Conversely, the health gains derived from national wealth appear to be maximized when policies, and the institutions which support them, are designed to universalize access to the resources needed to survive and thrive. In these societies, the emphasis is on providing a network of publicly funded services of sufficient range and scale to reduce inequalities in access to clean water and sanitation, income and food, education and health care. It is a policy approach which, in Sen's terms, seeks to enhance people's capabilities and to reduce inequalities in 'what people can be and what they can do' (UNDP, 2005: 51).

But it is a policy approach which middle-income and low-income countries have found increasingly hard to sustain. A major reason is the particular form that international economic integration has taken in recent decades (Box 5.2). Since the 1970s, globalization has become 'shorthand for global capitalism' (Birdsall, 2006: 22), with trade liberalization and financial deregulation enabling companies based in high-income countries to extend their reach into the economies, and the populations, of poorer countries. Global financial institutions, like the World Bank, International Monetary Fund

---

**Box 5.2**

---

'Globalisation is at present being shaped and defined within the specific discourse of market liberalism. Implicitly, it is a discourse that encourages views about the limits of government and the retreat from the public space.' (Mullard, 2004: xiii)

---

and World Trade Organization, have played an important role by negotiating what are called 'structural adjustment programmes' with poorer countries, often as a condition of financial aid and debt rescheduling (CSDH, 2005; Labonte and Schrecker, 2006; Sáinz, 2006). Actively promoted through the 1980s and 1990s, the programmes required that domestic markets were opened up to foreign investment and public expenditure was cut, with private companies taking over what were formerly publicly provided services (Box 5.3).

The effects of structural adjustment and of global capitalism more broadly, on low- and middle-income countries are matters of continuing controversy. But some broad consequences are apparent. There is general agreement that market-oriented policies, like the privatization of public services, tax reforms and financial liberalization, have squeezed the 'policy space' for national and sub-national governments to invest in redistributive policies. Thus, for example, structural adjustment programmes have been associated with cuts in food subsidies, reduced investment in sanitation and clean water supplies, and the introduction of fees for what were previously free health services (Whitehead *et al.*, 2001; CSDH, 2005; Homodes and Ugalde, 2005; Labonte and Schreker, 2005). There is evidence, too, of widening income inequalities. It appears that the benefits of economic growth are disproportionately concentrated in a small urban elite rather than distributed more widely across poorer and richer groups (Cornia, 2001). As one example,

---

**Box 5.3**

---

'The form and direction of changes undertaken as part of structural adjustment programs are in most respects identical to the market-oriented policy shifts that comprise a key element of globalization more generally . . . [For example] reduction of subsidies for basic items of consumption such as food, rapid removal of barriers to imports and foreign direct investment, reductions in state expenditures, particularly on social programmes such as health, education, water/ sanitation and housing, and rapid privatization of state-owned enterprises.' (Labonte and Schrecker, 2006: 18 and 16–17)

Box 5.4 summarizes the equity effects of economic transformation in Latin America.

---

**Box 5.4**

'Far-reaching economic and social changes . . . took place during the period 1980–2003. This period of transformation saw large-scale foreign actors gradually increase their economic and political power in Latin America, with negative consequences for domestic economies, especially in terms of increasing income inequality and rising poverty . . . Historically, Latin America has shown the worst income distribution of the world's regions. This situation deteriorated further in the 1980s and 1990s . . . [and] the percentage of the population in poverty in Latin America was higher in 2004 (44.0 per cent) than in 1980 (40.5 per cent).' (Sáinz, 2006: 1, 14 and 12)

---

'Outlier' countries like Sri Lanka have not been immune to the structural adjustment process. However, at least until the early 2000s, its health sector appeared to have been relatively protected from the outsourcing of services to the private sector and the introduction of user fees (Mills *et al.*, 2001). In India, the structural adjustment programme has been seen to have more far-reaching effects, with resources directed away from primary health care towards private hospitals and a sharp rise in the costs of health care, particularly for poorer groups (Qadeer, 2000; Thankappen, 2001). Analyses suggest that the programme has impacted negatively on Kerala, making it hard for the Indian state to sustain the principle of universal access to health care and threatening the survival of its redistributive model of welfare (Kutty, 2001; Thankappen, 2001). As this suggests, politics and policies matter for people's health. It is a theme to which the chapter returns after a brief consideration of health inequalities within countries.

## 5.3 Socio-economic inequalities in health within countries

Inequalities in health are evident within both poorer and richer societies. Figure 5.3 provides an indication of these inequalities in poorer societies. It focuses on under–5 mortality, and takes household income as its measure of socio-economic position. Figure 5.3 includes a middle-income country, South Africa (per capita GDP of $3500 in 2003), and three low-income countries: Ghana, one of the poorest countries in the world ($350), India ($550) and Nicaragua ($750) (UNDP, 2005). The steepness of the socio-economic gradient varies, with death rates falling much more rapidly with rising household

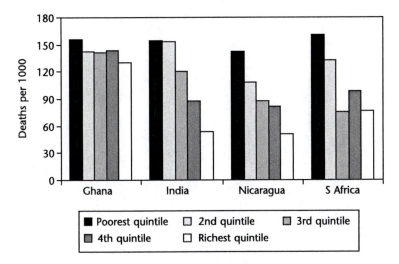

**Figure 5.3**  Under-5 mortality (deaths per 1000 live births) by income quintile in Ghana, India, Nicaragua and South Africa

*Source:* Gwatkin *et al.*, 2000, table 1 (India); Wagstaff, 2000, table 4 (Ghana, Nicaragua and South Africa)

income in India, Nicaragua and South Africa than in Ghana. But in all four countries, death rates are at their highest in the poorest households.

In rich societies, overall standards of health are much, much higher. But high overall standards mask the unequal distribution of health between more and less advantaged groups. Figure 5.4 captures patterns in the UK. Focusing on England and again using household income to measure socio-economic position, it maps the social gradients in long-term illnesses which restrict everyday activities across a range of minority ethnic groups (impairment and disability are discussed in Chapter 2, section 2.3 and ethnicity in Chapter 4, sections 4.1 and 4.2). The gradients are evident for men and women in all groups, with higher overall rates of limiting long-term illness in some groups (for example, Black Caribbean) than others (for example, Chinese).

Table 5.2 looks beyond England, and presents evidence of the unequal distribution of health in other European countries. Socio-economic position is measured by education and health by self-assessed health. Table 5.2 takes the rates of poor health in the most advantaged group (post-secondary education) as the reference category against which the rates in the most disadvantaged group (up to lower secondary education) are compared (see Chapter 2, section 2.5 for an explanation of relative inequalities in health). In England for example, the rates of poor health are three times higher among men in poorer circumstances compared with those in better circumstances; for women, rates are 2.7 times higher. Differences in the design of the studies

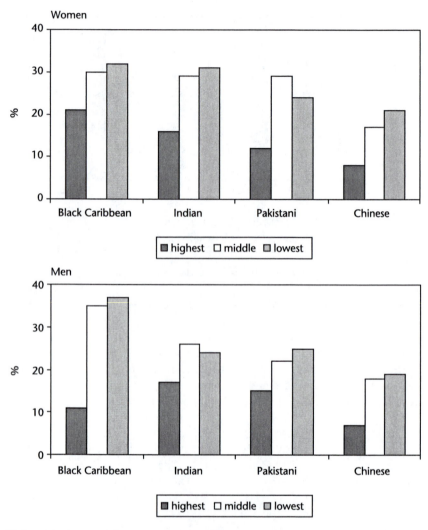

**Figure 5.4** Rates of limiting longstanding illness by equivalized household income tertile within minority ethnic groups, England, 1999

*Source:* Erens *et al.*, 2001, table 2.4

means that the magnitude of health inequalities in different countries cannot be directly compared: for example, it cannot be concluded that inequalities in England are larger than in Germany but similar to those found in Austria. But the broad picture is clear: across Europe, poorer circumstances are consistently associated with poorer health (Mackenbach, 2005a). It is a pattern repeated in the USA and Canada, as well as in Australia and New Zealand

**Table 5.2**   Socio-economic inequalities in self-assessed health in Europe in the 1990s: odds of poor health among men and women aged 25–69 years in the most disadvantaged group compared with the most advantaged group

|  | Men | Women |
|---|---|---|
| England | 3.08 | 2.66 |
| W. Germany | 1.76 | 1.91 |
| Finland | 2.99 | 3.29 |
| Sweden | 2.37 | 3.06 |
| Norway | 2.30 | 2.84 |
| Denmark | 2.16 | 3.00 |
| Netherlands | 2.81 | 2.12 |
| Austria | 3.22 | 2.67 |
| Italy | 2.94 | 2.55 |
| Spain | 2.58 | 3.10 |

*Note:* poor health based on a self-assessment of health as fair, poor or very poor.

*Source:* reproduced with permission from Kunst *et al.* (2005) *International Journal of Epidemiology* (April 2005) Oxford University Press.

(Elo and Preston, 1996; Turrell and Mathers, 2001; Blakely *et al.*, 2002; Wilkins *et al.*, 2002).

As this brief summary indicates, health is unequally distributed in both higher- and lower-income societies. However, poorer people fare better in some countries than others. For instance, the USA is much richer than the UK, with a GDP per person dwarfing that of its transatlantic neighbour. But socio-economic disadvantage is associated with much higher rates of ill health in the richer USA than in the poorer UK. As one example, in a study of 55 to 64-year-olds, using years of schooling and household income to measure socio-economic position, rates of diabetes among those in the most disadvantaged group were twice as high in the USA (over 14 per cent) as in the UK (7 per cent) (Banks *et al.*, 2006). Marked contrasts are evident, too, within high-income countries in Europe. Figure 5.5 focuses on four such countries with per capita incomes in 2001 which varied between $24,000 (England and Wales, and Sweden) and $32,000 (Ireland). Figure 5.5 gives the probability of a man in a manual group dying between the ages of 45 and 65. The probability of premature death is appreciably lower in Sweden and Norway (20 per cent) than in England and Wales (24 per cent) and Ireland (29 per cent). Thus, if a working-class man's aim was to reach retirement and he could chose where he lived, he would opt for Sweden or Norway in preference to England and Wales, or Ireland (Lundberg and Lahelma, 2001).

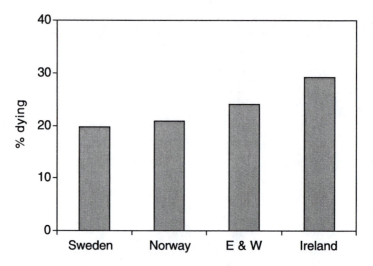

**Figure 5.5**   Probability of dying (percentage) between the age of 45 and 65 for men in manual social classes

*Source:* Kunst *et al.*, 1998, table 7

## 5.4 Socio-economic inequalities in health over time

Industrial expansion took off in Britain in the early nineteenth century. It was largely unregulated and concentrated in fast growing cities like Manchester, Liverpool, Birmingham and Glasgow (Box 5.5). Death rates in these cities increased sharply, prompting a mortality crisis which kept national life expectancy at around 40 years from 1800 to 1870 (Szreter and Mooney, 1998).

---

**Box 5.5**

'The development of factory production meant that workers were deprived of the opportunity to sell their labour on a relatively informal basis in dispersed geographical locations. The newly emerging wage workers were forced to migrate to the cities in order to work . . . by the deterioration of conditions in the countryside. As a consequence, towns expanded with enormous speed . . . In the decade from 1821–31 for example, the population of Manchester and Salford rose by 47 per cent, that of Bradford by 78 per cent and that of West Bromwich by 60 per cent. The standard of most housing was atrocious without clean water and effective sanitation.' (Doyal, 1979: 49–50)

The major causes of death were linked to poor sanitation and overcrowding. They included communicable diseases like tuberculosis, cholera and diphtheria, together with infant diarrhoea which, while recorded in official records as the precipitating cause of death, was typically infectious and parasitic in origin (Preston *et al.*, 1972; Wrigley *et al.*, 1997). In mid-nineteenth-century Britain, one child in five died before their fifth birthday (Farr, 1885).

High mortality rates were associated with marked inequalities in the health of rich and poor. For example in the 1860s, death rates among children aged 0–5 years stood at 460 per 1000 in poor cities like Liverpool and 175 per 1000 in prosperous districts like Hampstead on the outskirts of London (Farr, 1885). These inequalities in child mortality were reflected in inequalities in life expectancy. Figure 5.6 maps the socio-economic gradient in average age of death using occupational categories which reflected the social hierarchy of Victorian Britain. It lacks the precision expected of the UK's current socio-economic classifications (see Chapter 4, section 4.3). Nonetheless, it captures the unequal life chances of 'the three great classes of inhabitants: the wealthy, the tradespeople, and the artisans and labourers' (Lancet Editorial, 1843: 660). It highlights, too, the greater risk of early death for inhabitants of industrial centres like Manchester rather than for the populations of more provincial cities like York.

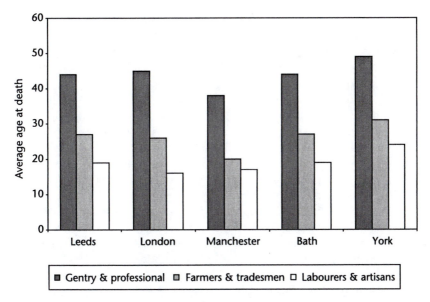

**Figure 5.6** Average age at death by the social class: Leeds, London (Bethnal Green), Manchester, Bath and York, 1838–41

*Source:* Lancet Editorial, 1843; Royal Commission on the Health of Towns, 1845

From the 1870s, survival rates improved and life expectancy in Britain at last started to rise. Behind the health gain was a decline in mortality from communicable diseases, a pattern evident in other early industrializing countries like the Netherlands (Mackenbach, 1996). At first the rise in life expectancy was modest, climbing from 41 years in 1870 to 47 years in 1900. Across the early decades of the twentieth century, the upward trend was steeper, with life expectancy reaching 58 years by 1921; by 1951, it stood at 65 years (Preston et al., 1972). The improvement in life expectancy among the non-combatant population was particularly marked during the war decades of 1910–20 and 1940–50. Six years was added to life expectancy between 1910 and 1920, with a further six-year increase between 1940 and 1950 (Preston et al., 1972).

The reasons for the increase in life expectancy have been much debated (see McKeown, 1979; Szreter, 1988; Winter, 1988; Mackenbach, 1996), but is widely agreed that better living conditions for the urban poor were a major factor. Better conditions were underpinned by a combination of rising real wages and environmental improvements, for example, in municipal public health, housing, factory safety and welfare services.

For the 1870–1910 period, the environmental changes included the development of integrated sewerage systems and piped clean water, improved housing conditions and improvements in the quality and regulation of the food supply (McKeown, 1979; Szreter, 1988; Doran and Whitehead, 2004). During 1910–20 and 1940–50, wartime welfare measures have been identified as particularly important in improving conditions for working-class families. In the 1940s, for example, the government intervened to stabilize the cost of, and to equalize access to, necessities through price controls, food subsidies and food rationing. At the same time, it extended welfare benefits and strengthened people's legal entitlement to health care (Seers, 1951; Titmuss, 1958). As Richard Titmuss notes, these measures 'universalised public provision for certain basic needs' (1958: 83). Tax changes further contributed to a levelling up of living standards of poorer households while holding down incomes of richer households (Seers, 1951). In turn, higher and more equitable living standards, and higher and more equitable nutritional standards in particular, contributed to the rapid improvement in life expectancy in the two 'war decades' (Hammond, 1951; Winter, 1988).

Historical analyses suggest that advances in medical care made a relatively small contribution to the rapid decline in mortality in the late nineteenth and early twentieth centuries. From the 1950s, medical care played a larger role in improving health, both in the UK and in other high-income countries (Mackenbach et al., 1988; Mackenbach, 1996). The middle decades of the twentieth century saw major advances in the treatment of infectious and chronic diseases (Tunstall-Pedoe et al., 2000; Bunker, 2001). They saw, too, the expansion of health-care systems in many high-income societies, funded through taxation (as in the UK and Sweden, for example) or by compulsory payroll deductions (the model adopted in Germany and France) (Esping-Andersen, 1993). A major aim of these different systems was to widen access to quality care, a vision strongly articulated in the UK's National Health Service (NHS). Launched in 1948, it was, as the Minister of Health Aneurin Bevan evocatively put it, about 'universalising the best' (quoted in Webster, 2001: 171). As the information leaflet distributed to every home made clear, 'everyone – rich or poor, man, woman or child – can use it or any part of it' (Box 5.6). Like the NHS, the health-care systems established in other high-income countries served to widen access to the new and more effective therapies, thus increasing their impact on people's health.

The 150-year improvement in life expectancy in Britain has been associated with a narrowing of absolute inequalities in health. In other high-income societies, too, improvements in population health have reduced the gap in rates of ill health between socio-economic groups. However, relative inequalities in health – differences in the risk of death in poorer groups compared with better-off groups – have proved to be more enduring. Box 5.7 summarizes the patterns in Europe.

It is a pattern captured in trends for infant mortality in England and Wales. Figure 5.7 is based on the Registrar General's class classification, with children born within marriage classified by their father's occupation (see Chapter 4,

---

**Box 5.6**

'Your National Health Service . . . will provide you with all medical, dental and nursing care. Everyone – rich or poor, man, woman or child – can use it or any part of it. There are no charges, except for a few special items. There are no insurance qualifications. But it is not a "charity". You are all paying for it, mainly as taxpayers, and it will relieve your money worries in time of illness.' (Front page of the NHS leaflet produced for the Ministry of Health in 1948, reproduced in Webster, 2001: 171)

---

**Box 5.7**

'Since the nineteenth century the magnitude of socioeconomic inequalities in mortality certainly declined in absolute terms: owing to the general decline in mortality the absolute differences in mortality between those with a high and those with a low socioeconomic position has become smaller. It is less clear whether relative inequalities have also declined: relative risks of dying for those in a low rather than a high socioeconomic position have remained remarkably stable.' (Mackenbach et al., 2002: 3)

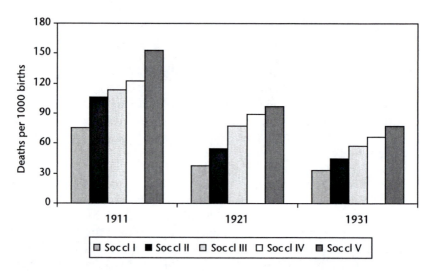

**Figure 5.7** Infant mortality by social class of father (deaths per 1000 live births within marriage) in early twentieth-century Britain

*Source:* Titmuss, 1943, table II

section 4.3). Figure 5.7 captures the improvement in this key dimension of health between 1911 and 1931 in all social classes. The improvement in the 'war decade' from 1911 to 1921 was particularly marked. The downward trend in infant mortality brought a narrowing of the *absolute* gap: this shrank from 77 deaths per 1000 live births in 1911 to 44 deaths per 1000 in 1931 (Box 5.8). But while absolute differences shrank, *relative* differences remained pronounced. As in 1911, children born into the poorest circumstances in the 1930s were still twice as likely to die before their first birthday as children in the best-off families. As a check on these findings, Richard Titmuss reanalysed the data to adjust for shortcomings in the 1911 classification of social class. He confirmed the patterns captured in Figure 5.7 (Titmuss, 1943).

---

**Box 5.8**

In 1911, infant mortality rates stood at 153 per 1000 among children born into the poorest circumstances (social class V) and 76 per 1000 among children born into best circumstances (social class I): an absolute difference in death rates of 77 deaths per 1000 per year (153 – 77 = 76).

By 1931, infant mortality rates had fallen in all social classes, to 77 per 1000 in social class V and 33 per 1000 in social class I: an absolute difference of 44 deaths per 1000 per year (77 – 33 = 44). (Registrar General, 1913)

This pattern – of persisting relative gaps despite narrowing absolute ones – is evident for many dimensions of health. But the pattern is not ubiquitous. For example, in England and Wales, both absolute and relative inequalities in male mortality appear to have narrowed in the 1920s and 1930s (Pamuk, 1985). Conversely, between the 1970s and the 1990s, inequalities in male mortality widened in both absolute and relative terms (Drever *et al.*, 1996).

## 5.5 Conclusions

The chapter has provided a brief review of health inequalities across place and over time. From this review, some common themes emerge.

First is the enduring association between greater wealth and better health: globally, nationally and historically. Those in the poorest conditions have the poorest health. Better-off groups enjoy better health than the poorest groups – but fail to achieve the standard of health enjoyed by those occupying the most privileged positions. This social gradient is evident in the patterning of health across rich and poorer countries (Figures 5.1 and 5.2, Table 5.1), as well as between richer and poorer groups within countries (Figures 5.3–5.7, Table 5.2).

The chapter's brief review brings out a second theme. While the mechanisms underlying these persisting inequalities are complex, policies emerge as important. Thus, across countries and over time, the relationship between wealth and health appears to be mediated by what national governments do – and, increasingly, what global agencies do – with the process and the proceeds of economic growth. Policies which underwrite people's living standards appear to be particularly important in protecting people's health, and protecting the health of poorer groups especially.

This second theme – that policies matter – widens the framework for understanding people's unequal lives. As noted in Chapters 3 and 4, it argues against a focus only on individuals and households, the units which form the primary unit of data collection and analysis in social epidemiology and health research. It directs our attention as well to the societal and global level. State-level and sub-national policies regulate the operation of markets, by protecting employment and working conditions, controlling prices and distributing essential resources. But, at the same time, nations are increasingly units of a larger global economic system currently run on free-market principles. The evidence suggests that today's global policies constrain what nations, and especially what poorer nations, can do to promote social and health equity.

The next chapter extends the review of health inequalities by examining the unequal patterning of health across changes in the major causes of death. Again, the evidence points to the importance of people's social conditions for their health, and thus the role that policy can play in narrowing inequalities in living standards and life chances.

# 6 Health inequalities across changes in disease

## 6.1 Introduction

Chapter 5 set the unequal distribution of health in a global, national and historical perspective. Building on this overview, Chapter 6 explores the persistence of inequalities across changes in the diseases which kill: evident when infectious diseases are the big killers, and re-emerging again when chronic diseases take over as the major cause of death.

The chapter begins by discussing the rise of chronic disease as the major cause of death in high-income societies, a pattern now being repeated on a global scale. It then turns to consider the increasing association between chronic disease and socio-economic disadvantage. It discusses some key risk factors, pointing to changes in food and tobacco consumption as well as increases in obesity, both within the UK and globally. The concluding section revisits the themes identified in Chapter 5, noting again the role of policy in steering countries through the process of social and economic change.

## 6.2 Socio-economic inequalities in health across changes in causes of death

In high-income societies like Britain, economic growth has been associated with a long-term decline in mortality and consequent improvement in life expectancy. With more people living longer, Britain's population increased rapidly, climbing from 37 million in 1900 to 49 million in 1950 and 57 million today (Hicks and Allen, 1999).

The shift from an agrarian economy to one based on manufacturing and, more recently, on service industries, has also been accompanied by changes in the diseases which kill: in what epidemiologists call the 'cause-structure of mortality'. There has been a shift from communicable diseases to non-communicable diseases as the major causes of death. These non-communicable diseases typically develop through long-term exposure to risk factors. In part, their increasing importance is the consequence of the decline in child mortality and the increasing proportion of the population living long enough to die from 'slow-burn' diseases.

In addition, and more importantly, it reflects a rapid increase in deaths from circulatory disease and cancer across a period in which the death toll from infectious diseases was falling rapidly. Figure 6.1 plots the trend in these broad categories of disease for Britain across the twentieth century. While patterns for these broad categories are clear, changes in disease classification and in coding practices for cause of death mean that it is difficult to map trends for specific causes of death with precision (see Chapter 2, section 2.2). However, there is considerable evidence that deaths from ischemic heart disease and lung cancer reached epidemic proportions. Analyses suggest that ischemic heart disease was already a major cause of death by the 1920s, with mortality rates rising rapidly to peak in the 1970s for both men and women before falling (Charlton and Murphy, 1997). Lung cancer mortality increased from 1910, with an earlier and sharper increase among men than women. Death rates have been declining among men since the 1970s; among women, the upward trend in death rates from lung cancer continued to the early 1990s and is declining only gradually (Charlton and Murphy, 1997; Doll *et al.*, 1997; Griffiths and Brock, 2003).

The concept of an 'epidemiologic transition' was coined by Abdel Omran in the 1970s to describe the change in the cause-structure of mortality in early industrializing countries of northern Europe. Also referred to as the

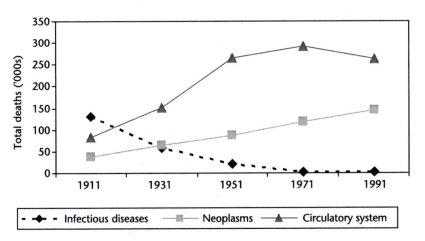

**Figure 6.1** Total deaths from infectious diseases, neoplasms and circulatory system, Britain, 1911–91

*Source:* Charlton and Murphy, 1997, table 4.4a

'epidemiological transition', Omran characterized it as (1971: 736–7): 'A long-term shift in mortality and disease patterns whereby the pandemics of infection are gradually displaced by degenerative and man-made diseases as the chief form of morbidity and primary cause of death.'

Britain provides an example of this long-term shift (Figure 6.1). Box 6.1 maps the changing proportion of deaths attributed to infectious and parasitic diseases and to cancer and circulatory disease over the last 130 years.

There is evidence of Omran's epidemiologic transition in countries which have more recently shifted from rural and agrarian to urban and industrial (Box 6.2). In low- and middle-income countries, communicable diseases remain the leading cause of child deaths. But non-communicable diseases now account for more than 50 per cent of adult deaths in all regions except south Asia and sub-Saharan Africa (Lopez *et al.*, 2006). In low-, middle- and high-income countries, ischemic heart disease and cerebrovascular disease (of which stroke is the major example) are the leading causes of adult deaths (Lopez *et al.*, 2006).

However, this broad picture masks more complex patterns. Many poorer

---

**Box 6.1**

In 1880, cancer and circulatory disease were identified as the cause of 10 per cent of deaths. By 1900, the proportion had reached 25 per cent and had climbed to 60 per cent by 1950. The proportion peaked at over 70 per cent in the 1970s and 1980s. In 2005, over 60 per cent of deaths had cancer and circulatory disease as their underlying cause. (Preston *et al.*, 1972; Charlton and Murphy, 1997; Hicks and Allen, 1999; Health Statistics Quarterly, 2006b)

---

**Box 6.2**

'Between 1900 and 2000, Mexico evolved from a rural, agricultural economy with just over 13 million inhabitants and a high proportion of children to a predominantly urban one with over 90 million inhabitants mainly aged 15 to 44, and primarily employed in the least productive, worst-paid activities in the tertiary sector . . . The profile of the causes of death also experienced significant changes. Records . . . from 1922 show, at that time, people dying mainly from pneumonia and influenza, diarrhoea and enteritis, fever, whooping cough and small pox. At the end of the century, nearly half of all deaths were due to cardiovascular disease, malign tumors, diabetes mellitus and car accidents.' (Carolina and Gustava, 2003: 543)

countries are not following the path taken by high-income nations. 'Pandemics of infection' are persisting alongside a rapid increase in 'degenerative and man-made diseases'. Particularly in countries where HIV/AIDs and malaria kills large numbers, the transition is leading to what has been called a 'double burden' of disease, with high rates of acute, infectious diseases persisting alongside an increase in chronic, non-infectious diseases (Box 6.3). Injuries (particularly from road traffic accidents and violence) are also a significant cause of premature death in many low and middle countries, suggesting that they face not a double, but a triple, burden of disease (Lopez *et al.*, 2006).

Little is known about the socio-economic patterning of deaths from chronic disease in high-income countries in the early stages of the epidemiologic transition. Changing diagnostic practices make firm conclusions even harder to draw. But there is evidence to suggest that the familiar class gradients were often absent, with mortality rates either similar across socio-economic groups or higher among more advantaged groups. Thus British analyses of lung cancer mortality among men suggest that there was little association with social class in the early decades of the twentieth century (Townsend and Davidson, 1982). For heart disease, mortality rates from coronary artery disease were higher among men in social classes I and II than in social classes III, IV and V from 1911 to 1951 (Davey Smith, 1997). As the century progressed and deaths from chronic disease increased, the socio-economic profile started to change. By the 1960s, death rates among men from lung cancer and coronary artery disease were higher in social classes IV and V than in I and II (Townsend and Davidson, 1982; Davey Smith, 1997). The familiar gradients have become more marked over time: as Figure 6.2 suggests, the so-called 'diseases of affluence' are increasingly diseases of poverty.

Figure 6.2 points to falling death rates from chronic diseases in all socio-economic groups. But as it makes clear, the rate of decline has been faster among more advantaged groups. It is these steepening gradients in the 'big killers' which underlie the increase in inequalities in all-cause mortality in the UK (Marmot and McDowall, 1986; Drever and Whitehead, 1997; DoH, 2005). A similar picture is evident in other high-income countries: more

---

**Box 6.3**

'A feature of the current global health status picture is the "double burden" of disease. Countries that are still struggling with old and new infectious-disease epidemics must now deal with the emerging epidemics of chronic non-communicable diseases such as heart disease, stroke, diabetes and cancer.' (Sen and Bonita, 2000: 580)

Lung cancer

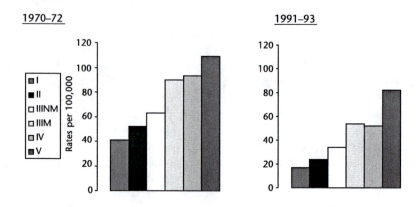

Ischemic heart disease

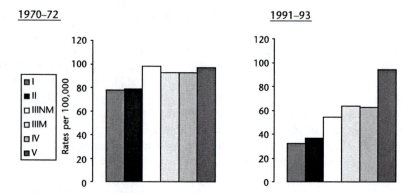

**Figure 6.2**   European standardised mortality rate by social class, men aged 20–64, lung cancer and ischemic heart disease

*Source:* Drever and Bunting, 1997, table 8.6

rapid declines in death rates in higher socio-economic groups are widening inequalities in health (Box 6.4).

## 6.3  Social patterning of risk factors for chronic disease

Major causes of death like ischemic heart disease and lung cancer are linked to a cluster of behavioural and physiological factors. The cluster includes cigarette smoking, a diet high in saturated fats, sugar and refined food, physical

---

**Box 6.4**

---

'Mortality differences between socio-economic groups have widened in many Western European countries during the last three decades of the 20th century . . . The explanation of this disturbing phenomenon is only partly known. One aspect should certainly be taken into account, however, is that this widening of the relative gap in death rates is generally the result of a difference between socio-economic groups in the speed of the mortality decline. While mortality declined in all socio-economic groups, the decline has been proportionately faster in the higher socio-economic groups than in the lower.' (Mackenbach, 2005a: 8)

---

inactivity and overweight and obesity. These factors figure prominently among the leading global risk factors for mortality (Lopez *et al.*, 2006). Nine in ten deaths from lung cancer – the leading global cause of cancer deaths – are attributed to smoking, a habit also implicated in other chronic diseases. Smoking is estimated to cause 28 per cent of deaths in high-income countries and 20 per cent worldwide. Being overweight and obese elevates the risk of diabetes and circulatory disease, and have been identified as second only to smoking as the leading cause of preventable disease and death in high-income countries (USDHHS, 2001) and, along with smoking, among 'the most important global health risk factors' (Chopra and Darnton-Hill, 2004: 1558).

In pre-industrial and low-income countries, the prevalence of these risk factors has historically been low. Only a minority of the population have access to manufactured cigarettes and processed foods, and obesity is rare. As countries get richer, more people smoke cigarettes, diets change and rates of obesity and being overweight start to climb, trends often first evident in the expanding urban middle class. As prevalence of these risk factors increase, their socio-economic profile changes. How can these complex patterns be understood?

### Changing societies, new risk factors

A key dynamic appears to be the disruption, and consequent transformation, of traditional food systems, forms of tobacco use and patterns of physical activity through the process of economic change. Industrialization has typically taken the form of rapid urban expansion, with the rural population migrating to towns and cities to work in factories and offices. In the process, traditional ways of living and working have given way to ones characterized by low energy expenditure and by high consumption both of tobacco and of food products that undermine health.

Until the twentieth century, the dominant forms of *tobacco use* – like pipes, cigars, snuff and chewing tobacco – were not very palatable and were regulated by restrictive social norms (Goodman, 1993). In northern Europe and the USA, for example, it was considered inappropriate for women to use tobacco; among men, consumption levels were very low by twentieth century standards (Wald and Nicolaides-Bouman, 1991). But in the closing decades of the nineteenth century, a milder and more palatable medium for tobacco consumption was introduced. The new product could be produced cheaply for a mass market (Box 6.5) and, delivering nicotine more efficiently into the blood stream, was much more addictive. By the early twentieth century, manufactured cigarettes were displacing traditional tobacco products in both the USA and the UK, fuelling a rapid increase in tobacco consumption first among men and then among women (Graham, 1993). By the 1940s, 65 per cent of men and 40 per cent of women in the UK were smoking manufactured cigarettes (Wald and Nicolaides-Bouman, 1991).

As reliance on farming and farming-related industries has given way to manufacturing and service industries, the trends found in northern Europe have been repeated in southern Europe. Thus in the mid-decades of the twentieth century, men in France and Italy began to abandon traditional tobacco products in favour of manufactured cigarettes, a pattern followed in subsequent decades by Spain, Portugal and Greece (Lee, 1975; Nicolaides-Bouman *et al.*, 1993). Again, these countries have seen women follow men into the new cigarette market, fuelling a rapid increase in their rates of tobacco use since the 1970s (Graham, 1996).

While historical data for middle- and low-income countries are sparse, there is evidence to suggest that the patterns found in richer countries are being reproduced on a global scale. Traditional forms of tobacco use are more widely used by men, and it is men who appear to be leading the way into cigarette smoking. Since the 1970s, cigarette consumption has been rising rapidly in poorer countries – across decades in which it has been falling in high-income countries (Gajalakshmi *et al.*, 2000). The result is high rates of overall tobacco use among men. In China and India for example, studies

---

**Box 6.5**

'The story of cigarettes (in the US) begins in 1861 when James Bonsack patented a cigarette-making machine that manufactured up to forty times what the best skilled workers could produce by hand. Within a decade, the cost of producing a cigarette was reduced to one-sixth of what it had been. When James Buchanan Duke turned exclusively to machine production in 1885, he quickly saturated the American market. Production was no longer a problem: the only task was to sell.' (Studson, 1993: 185)

suggest that over 60 per cent of men are tobacco users (Gajalakshmi *et al.*, 2000; Sorensen *et al.*, 2005). High rates among men are also reported in countries in Latin America and Africa (UNDP, 2005).

Until the nineteenth century, countries produced and consumed *food products* locally, and largely independently of each other. Staple foods, and the diets they supported, therefore tended to be specific to the areas in which they originate (Sobal, 1999). These local diets were typically grain- and vegetable-based, with high consumption of fat-rich foods (like meat and dairy products) the preserve of the rich. As living standards rose in the early-industrializing countries of northern Europe and North America, both diets and their systems of production changed. Average consumption of fat-rich and energy-dense foods increased, and industries to produce, process and distribute these foods began to emerge. In today's low- and middle-income countries, there is evidence that higher consumption of fats and sugars is triggered at lower levels of national wealth and more directly in response to rapid urban growth. Dietary changes which extended over half a century in older industrial societies are taking place in poorer countries in less than a decade (Drewnowski and Popkin, 1997). The food industry has been implicated in this process, with domestic food systems initially developed for rich countries finding new markets among the much larger populations of low- and middle-income countries (Box 6.6). The result is a 'McDonaldization' and 'coca-colonization' of poorer countries (Sobal, 1999; Zimmet, 2000), in which buying and drinking Coke, and spending and eating at McDonalds, have become 'uniform and universal global experiences' (Mullard, 2004: 148).

Changes in diet, together with declines in physical activity, are implicated in the increase in overweight and obesity (defined in Box 6.7). As Jebb *et al.* note

---

**Box 6.6**

'Food advertising is rising in developing countries; it has tripled in South East Asia, for example. Within a few years of [its] introduction, 65% of the Chinese population recognised the brand name of Coca Cola . . . Mexicans now drink more Coca Cola than milk'. (Chopra and Darnton-Hill, 2004: 1558–9)

---

**Box 6.7**

The World Health Organization measures overweight and obesity by body mass index (BMI), by dividing a person's weight by their height and squaring the result (weight/height$^2$). A BMI of $\geq 25$ marks a person as overweight and one of $\geq 30$ defines them as obese (see WHO Expert Committee, 1995).

'it is now generally accepted that obesity develops in response to adverse environmental factors, which favour increased food consumption and decreased energy expenditure' (2003: 577). In response to these adverse environmental conditions, the prevalence of obesity in Britain doubled between 1980 and 2000 (Erens *et al.*, 2001). By the early 2000s, 67 per cent of men, 60 per cent of women and 25 per cent of children were overweight (Sproston and Primatesta, 2004; Jotangia *et al.*, 2005). Similar trends are reported in other high-income countries, including Australia and the USA (Chopra and Darnton-Hill, 2004; Hinde and Dixon, 2004). Rates of obesity and being overweight have also increased rapidly in middle- and low-income countries. In parts of the Middle East, north Africa and Latin America, prevalence of obesity among women is similar to, or above, those in the USA and the UK (Martorell *et al.*, 2000). A similar pattern is evident for childhood obesity, with trends in China and South Africa beginning to approach levels in the USA (Drewnowski and Popkin, 1997).

### Changing social gradients in risk factors

A century ago, cigarette smoking was a minority habit, even in high-income societies where the habit first took hold. While the evidence is limited, it suggests that it was young adults in privileged circumstances – affluent, well educated and city-living – who were the first to take up the new tobacco product (Graham, 1993; Hilton, 2000).

Figure 6.3 picks up the story for Britain from the late 1950s, when national surveys first began to collect information on tobacco use by social class. It combines a range of data sources to map trends in cigarette smoking among men and women in professional (social class I) and unskilled manual (social class V) groups. The range of data sources, together with changes in the measurement of socio-economic position, mean that Figure 6.3 can only give a very broad indication of these trends. Nonetheless, some features are clear. By the late 1950s, cigarette smoking was a widespread habit among both men and women, and one without a clear class profile. However, prevalence rates in higher socio-economic groups were already falling. Interestingly, the downward trend was in train before the link between smoking and lung cancer was being actively disseminated – and several decades before the health risks of smoking were widely communicated through media campaigns and advice leaflets (Doll and Hill, 1950; Berridge and Loughlin, 2005). The downward trend through the 1950s, 1960s and early 1970s was not matched among poorer groups. As Figure 6.3 indicates, the prevalence of cigarette smoking in these groups has fallen since but the rate of decline has been modest.

These changing patterns of smoking mean that, in the UK as in other high-income societies, buying and smoking cigarettes is no longer a cultural

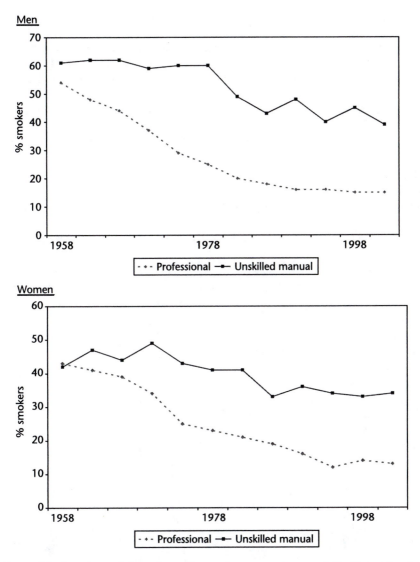

**Figure 6.3**  Prevalence of cigarette smoking among men and women in the highest (professional) and lowest (unskilled manual) socio-economic groups, Britain, 1958–2000

*Source:* Wald and Nicolaides-Bouman, 1991, table 5.2; ONS, 2001, table 8.8

signifier of class distinction. It has become, instead, a habit linked to class disadvantage. Today, this link emerges in adolescence, the life stage when smoking careers are established. As Figure 6.4 indicates, it is young people from disadvantaged backgrounds who are likely to smoke regularly and smoke more heavily by the age of 15. Poorer childhood circumstances and heavier smoking in adolescence have been found to influence subsequent smoking habits, with each factor reducing the chances of quitting and increasing the odds of remaining a smoker into middle age (Jefferis *et al.*, 2003).

The patterns characterizing the smoking epidemic in the UK are being played out elsewhere. In southern Europe for example, there is evidence that manufactured cigarettes were first incorporated into the lifestyles of the young urban middle class, with the class profile changing as the habit subsequently spread across the population (Graham, 1996; Cavelaars *et al.*, 2000; Huisman *et al.*, 2005). Today, cigarette smoking among men in southern Europe is more prevalent in lower than higher socio-economic groups (Cavelaars *et al.*, 2000; Huisman *et al.*, 2005). Among women, rates still tend to be higher in higher socio-economic groups; however, patterns among younger groups suggest that the socio-economic gradients which are so firmly entrenched in northern Europe are now emerging (Graham, 1996; Huisman *et al.*, 2005).

Less is known about the social patterning of tobacco use in middle- and low-income countries. The limited evidence suggests that traditional tobacco

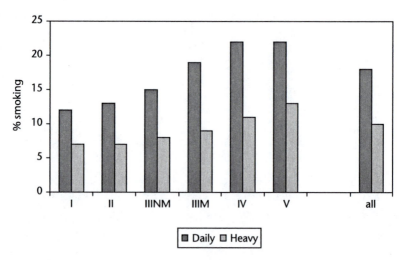

**Figure 6.4** Prevalence of daily and heavy smoking among young people aged 15 by parental social class, Scotland, 1999

*Source:* Sweeting and West, 2001, table 1

products are more widely used by poorer groups. In some countries, the uptake of cigarette smoking appears to follow trends found in high-income countries, with higher rates of cigarette smoking reported in higher socio-economic groups. For example, a study in the early 1990s in Mumbai (India) found that men in the highest educational and occupational groups had the highest rates of cigarette smoking (rates among women in all groups were very low) (Sorenson *et al.*, 2005). But an increasingly common pattern is for higher prevalence of cigarette smoking among poorer groups (Bobak *et al.*, 2000). Thus, studies in Malawi and Zambia suggest that it is poorer groups who first adopted the new tobacco product and that rates have remained higher in these groups (Pampel, 2005). As Pampel notes, historical changes in the socio-economic profile of cigarette smoking in high-income countries may not provide a model through which to understand the diffusion of cigarette smoking in low-income nations today.

The rapid rise of obesity has similarly been associated with changes in its social profile. In the UK, socio-economic inequalities in adult obesity were largely absent in the 1960s (Power *et al.*, 2003). However, among children, socio-economic gradients were already beginning to emerge for girls (Peckham *et al.*, 1983). As rates of childhood obesity have increased, socio-economic gradients have become evident among boys and steepened among girls, with the upward trend in obesity and being overweight more marked among children from poorer backgrounds (Kinra *et al.*, 2005; Stamatakis *et al.*, 2005). The patterns found for children are also evident among adults. As rates of adult obesity and being overweight have risen, the association between socio-economic disadvantage and excess body weight has strengthened (Wadsworth *et al.*, 2003). Again, the association tends to be stronger for women than men, a pattern repeated in other early-industrializing countries (Sobal and Stunkard, 1989; Sproston and Primatesta, 2004). In eastern European countries, and in southern European countries like Spain, Portugal and Greece, socio-economic gradients in obesity are now apparent among women; among men, the association between disadvantage and obesity again tends to be weaker (Cavelaars *et al.*, 1997; Molarius *et al.*, 2000).

Up until the late 1980s, positive socio-economic gradients in obesity were widely reported for low- and middle-income countries, with the highest rates among the most advantaged groups (Sobal and Stunkard, 1989; Wang, 2001). These positive gradients were evident for men, women and children. Greater access to food, lower energy expenditure and a high cultural value attached to a fat body shape were identified as explaining the link between social advantage and obesity. But the socio-economic profile of obesity appears to change in societies where economic growth is combined with rapid urbanization (Box 6.8). Again, these changes are often most marked among women. There is evidence that the positive association between wealth and obesity found in low-income societies flattens in low to

---

**Box 6.8**

---

'Growing rates of obesity in low and middle-income countries are still positively linked with higher household incomes. However, there are already instances in Latin America and in Caribbean countries where the poor are more likely to be obese than the rich . . . We predict that this inverse relationship between obesity and incomes will be found in more countries within a decade, particularly in countries characterised by large agglomerates of urban poor.' (Drewnowski and Popkin, 1997: 40)

---

middle-income countries before giving way to a negative association in upper middle-income countries, like Egypt, Mexico, Turkey and Brazil (Martorell *et al.*, 2000; Monteiro *et al.*, 2004).

## 6.4 Conclusions

Chapters 5 and 6 have provided an overview of the patterns of unequal health. What broad conclusions can be drawn from the review?

First, the chapters have pointed to rising life expectancy in many, but not all, societies. The patterns are complex but they suggest that improvements in people's living conditions underlie improvements in their life expectancy, with better conditions driving down death rates from causes linked to infection and nutrient-deficient diets, particularly among children. In societies which have experienced cumulative improvements in living conditions, each successive generation has a relative health advantage over the generation before.

Second, despite better living conditions and better health for the majority of the world's population, the review has uncovered persisting socio-economic gradients in health: between and within societies as well as over time. These gradients are evident when infectious diseases dominate the mortality statistics – and they re-emerge as non-communicable diseases take hold. As this suggests, socio-economic inequalities in health endure despite changes in the mechanisms through which disadvantage takes its toll on health. As Hertzman (2001) observes, 'the gradient effect is evident for virtually all the major diseases that affect health and wellbeing [and] . . . as the major diseases have changed over time, the gradient effect has replicated itself on new diseases as they have emerged' (2001: 46). What this means is that, at any point in time, children and adults in poorer circumstances are disproportionately exposed to the risk factors and diseases which drive death rates in the societies of which they are part.

Third, in tracing the persistence of health inequalities over time and across diseases, the chapters have drawn attention to the impact of economic change. In high-income societies, the twin processes of industrialization and urbanization triggered a century-long shift from infectious to chronic disease (the epidemiologic transition). Low- and middle-income countries are undergoing the shift from an agriculture-based to an industry-based economy in very different circumstances and on a highly condensed timescale. While evidence is limited, it suggests that the drive for economic growth is disrupting traditional food systems and, at the same time, increasing consumption of processed foods and manufactured cigarettes. As Carolina and Gustavo put it, 'traditional agricultural societies abruptly transformed into poor urban societies have left their members exposed to the lowest level of the modern industrial lifestyle from whose risks they are entirely unprotected' (2003: 542).

Underlying this abrupt transformation is a particular form of globalization. It is one which favours the integration of national economies into global systems for commodity production. Features include opening up poorer countries to powerful transnational corporations and reducing public sector provision of public health and welfare services. One consequence is that poorer countries can simultaneously provide new markets for manufactured tobacco and 'junk food' (energy dense, nutrient poor) and at the same time lack clean water and sewage disposal (De Beyer *et al.*, 2001; Leatherman and Goodman, 2005). For example, in Bangladesh, where smoking rates among men aged 35–49 stand at over 70 per cent, more than 80 per cent of the population live on less than US$2 a day and the majority of the population are without access to sanitation (Efroymson *et al.*, 2001; World Bank, 2003; SDNP, 2005).

An appreciation of economic contexts and economic forces leads to the fourth conclusion. Policies are important. The evidence reviewed in the chapters suggests that national and sub-national policies steer countries through economic change, and thus mediate the health and equity effects of rapid industrialization and urbanization. Thus, as Chapter 5 notes, low-income countries like Sri Lanka have secured higher levels of population health than their wealth would predict by using their limited national wealth for what Rawls calls primary social goods and for the public services which secure them, including sanitation and safe water, the provision of staple foods at affordable prices, education and health care. Conversely, high-income countries like the USA, which provide only the most basic of welfare safety nets, can find themselves paying the price through lower levels of population health than rich societies with more extensive welfare states.

# PART 3
# Understandings

Part 1 discussed what is meant by socio-economic inequalities in health, and the measures of health and socio-economic position that researchers use to capture these inequalities. Part 2 described the patterns revealed using the measures, noting the persistence of health inequalities across and within societies as well as across, and despite changes in, the diseases which kill. Together, Parts 1 and 2 provide the foundation on which to deepen our understanding of inequalities in people's socio-economic circumstances and their enduring association with inequalities in people's health.

This is the aim of the Part 3. It begins by discussing the conceptual frameworks that health researchers have developed to map the links between social and health inequalities. Chapter 7 notes that these frameworks highlight a web of causal pathways running from the social structure through social position to health. Chapters 8 and 9 address the 'upstream' end, and focus on the intersections between social structures and socio-economic position. They discuss research which is illuminating how inequalities in socio-economic position are reproduced across generations (from parent to child) and across people's lives (from childhood to adulthood). The chapters look in particular at the role of educational trajectories and domestic trajectories in this process. Chapter 10 looks 'downstream' from socio-economic position, investigating how inequalities in people's circumstances become embodied in their health. As in Part 2, the evidence reviewed in these chapters points to the importance of policy in influencing how unequal a society is. Chapter 11 explores this question directly. It highlights the extent to which socio-economic inequalities are policy sensitive, giving examples of how policies can and do make a difference to how unequal people's lives are. As in the earlier parts of the book, the UK is a major focus of analysis in Part 3.

# 7  Social determinants of health and health inequalities

## 7.1 Introduction

The chapters which make up Part 3 of the book are concerned with understanding why people's lives and people's health are so unequal. The conceptual and empirical foundations for this understanding have been laid down in Parts 1 and 2.

Part 1 provided the conceptual tools. It noted that the term 'health inequalities' is widely used to refer to inequalities in people's health which are linked to inequalities in their position in society. Socio-economic inequalities in health are therefore inequalities in health associated with people's unequal socio-economic positions. Chapter 3 discussed what social researchers mean by socio-economic position. The concept is generally seen to refer to people's position in the social structures through which economic resources and rewards – like jobs and earnings – are distributed. An individual's socio-economic position is therefore heavily dependent on their position in the labour market which, in turn, is influenced by their family background and their educational trajectory. Sociological research suggests that inequalities in these positions are produced and maintained as people make their way through their lives – and thus make their way from their natal family through the education system and into the labour market. Building on these conceptual chapters, Part 2 summarized empirical research on the association between people's socio-economic position and their health. It described how socio-economic inequalities in health were evident across place, time and major causes of death. The chapters pointed to the role of government policy in influencing the extent to which a country's wealth is used to level up people's socio-economic circumstances and equalize their access to health resources.

Part 3 deepens the analysis of social and health inequalities by looking more closely at how socio-economic and health inequalities are forged and maintained. Chapters 8 and 9 focus on the connections between social structures and social positions, reviewing research which sheds light on how inequalities in socio-economic position persist over time and across generations. Chapter 10 is concerned with how these persisting inequalities become 'written on the body' in the form of health inequalities. Chapter 11 explores the contribution of policy to moderating inequalities in people's circumstances.

This chapter provides an introduction to the three chapters by focusing on the conceptual frameworks which health researchers have developed to map the connections between social structures, social position and health. While these frameworks vary, they convey a common message. They make clear that factors lying beyond the reach of the health-care system are the primary influences on people's health and that, by implication, the unequal distribution of these factors is the principal cause of health inequalities. This central message is conveyed through the concept of the social determinants of health. Section 7.2 traces the recent history of the concept and its incorporation in public health policy. Section 7.3 discusses how it has been deployed in the frameworks developed by health researchers, noting how inequalities in the distribution of social determinants are implicit but integral to these frameworks. Section 7.4 discusses the pivotal position of social position in models of the social determinants of health and health inequalities.

## 7.2 The emerging focus on social determinants

In early industrializing countries like the UK, the public health profession played an important role in highlighting the human consequences of unregulated urban growth. Through the late nineteenth century, they argued for policies to improve the living and working conditions of the urban poor, including measures to secure safe drinking water and basic standards of sanitation and housing (Evans, 1978; Whitehead, 1997). But the early decades of the twentieth century saw a 'narrowing of public health's mandate' to individual level interventions and to health education in particular (Lewis, 1986: 6). As the century progressed and death rates from heart disease and cancer increased, the remit and resources for public health were squeezed still further, as governments turned to clinical medicine to tackle the chronic disease epidemic.

Against this backdrop, a series of influential critiques of health policy were published in the 1970s (for example, McKeown, 1971, 1979; Illich, 1975; McKinlay, 1975; Navarro, 1976; Doyal, 1979). The critics came from different disciplinary and professional backgrounds. Nonetheless, there was considerable common ground between them. The critics were united in the view that national and global health policy was too heavily weighted to clinical interventions for people who are ill and gave too little attention to the social conditions which keep people well. This shared conclusion rested on other points of agreement.

For example, all were critical of the influence exerted by the health-care industry over health policy and health expenditure. Thus John McKinlay noted that private and public spending was 'increasingly tied to the priorities of profit-making institutions' (McKinlay,1975: 8) and Ivan Illich argued that 'the medical establishment has become a major threat to health (which) . . . cannot but obscure the political conditions which render society unhealthy' (Illich, 1975: 11). There was general agreement, too, that the conditions which rendered people unhealthy lay, not in medicine, but in the social and material environment. It was a consensus informed by Thomas McKeown's historical analysis of the decline of mortality in England and Wales. He argued that 'the contribution of clinical medicine to the prevention of death and increase in the expectation of life in the past three centuries was smaller than that of other influences' (McKeown, 1979: 91). Among these 'other influences', he highlighted environmental improvements (see Box 7.1 and Chapter 5, section 5.4). There was therefore, as McKinlay put it, 'a case for refocusing upstream . . . away from those individuals and groups who are mistakenly held responsible for their (health) condition, toward a range of broader upstream political and economic forces' (1975: 7).

McKinlay's metaphor of 'upstream' and 'downstream' was inspired by a story told to him by the American sociologist Irving Zola. The story involved a doctor who was too busy jumping in and rescuing drowning people from a swiftly flowing river 'to see who the hell is upstream pushing them all in' (McKinlay, 1975: 7). In the story and McKinlay's analysis, 'downstream' therefore refers to medical care; 'upstream' to a wider and more powerful set of factors which shape people's health. Box 7.2 illustrates the recurrent emphasis on these upstream factors, variously referred to as the environment, living and working conditions and determinants beyond the health care system. It is this emphasis which is captured in the concept of the social determinants of health. In line with Doyal's definition (Box 7.2), the concept often refers specifically to people's living and working conditions. Thus the WHO's

---

**Box 7.1**

'The main reason for the decline [in mortality from mid-nineteenth century], in order of time and magnitude, were (a) an improvement in the standard of living, particularly of nutrition, (b) hygienic measures from about 1870, and (c) prevention and treatment of disease in the individual from the second quarter of the present [twentieth] century . . . Effective prevention and treatment of disease in the individual were delayed until the second quarter of the twentieth century and have been less significant than any of the other major influences'. (McKeown, 1971: 32–3, and 45)

---

**Box 7.2**

'Analysis of disease trends shows that the environment is the primary determinant of the state of general health of any population. Food, housing, working conditions, neighbourhood cohesion . . . play the decisive role in how healthy grown-ups feel and at what age adults tend to die.' (Illich, 1975: 17)

'The determinants of health . . . result from environmental influences.' (McKeown, 1979: 117)

'[We need to] make sense of the impact of living and working conditions, and patterns of social and economic relationships, on the health of individuals and groups . . . A critical analysis of the social determinants of health and illness and of the role of medicine is now emerging.' (Doyal, 1979: 296 and 11)

'The determinants of health which lie outside the health care system . . . may be quantitatively very significant for the overall health of modern populations . . . The health of individuals and populations is affected by their health care, but also by other factors as well.' (Evans and Stoddart, 1990: 1355 and 1360)

---

Commission on the Social Determinants of Health (CSDH) states that 'people's health largely depends on the social conditions in which they live and work – the social determinants of health' (CSDH, 2006: 3). However, the concept tends to have a looser meaning in public health policy, with more emphasis given to behavioural influences on health.

The 1970s' critiques quickly made their way into debates about public health policy. An early example was a report by Canada's Minister of National Health and Welfare, Marc Lalonde (Box 7.3). The report referred explicitly to McKeown's argument that social policies, not medical interventions, hold the key to improving people's health. It goes on to note that, with medical care taking the lion's share of the health budget, governments were failing to address 'the underlying causes of mortality and morbidity' (Lalonde, 1974: 13).

---

**Box 7.3**

'[F]or . . . environmental and behavioural threats to health, the organized health care system can do little more than serve as a catchment net for the victims. Physicians, surgeons, nurses and hospitals spend much of their time in treating ills caused by adverse environmental factors and behavioural risks.' (Lalonde, 1974: 5)

---

The Lalonde report was part of a wider political re-engagement with public health, a re-engagement which found its most visionary expression in the *Health for All (HFA)* charter of the late 1970s. This committed national governments and the World Health Organization (WHO) to secure a decent level of health for all by the year 2000 (WHO, 1981, 1998). Improving the health of poorer groups was recognized to be central to this vision, to be achieved through universal access to basic services, including primary care. To support the WHO's *HFA* equity agenda, Göran Dahlgren and Margaret Whitehead prepared a strategy paper outlining 'the main influences on health' (Box 7.4). These influences were captured in a simple model consisting of a set of concentric arcs. In a revised and more detailed form, the model has become the most widely known depiction of the social determinants of health. Figure 7.1 gives the most recent version of their rainbow model (Dahlgren and Whitehead, 2006).

Through the 1990s, the *HFA* agenda was slowly influencing national policy-making. Governments began to confront the fact that, even in high-income societies, there was health for some, not health for all. It was a realization which prompted a re-evaluation and a widening of the goals of health policy. By the early 2000s, reducing health inequalities had been placed alongside improving population health as a core policy goal in the UK, Ireland, the Netherlands and Sweden; in Finland, health equity has been an avowed goal of public heath policy since the 1980s (Secretary of State for Health, 1999; DHSSPS, 2000; DHC, 2001; MSAH, 2001). Beyond Europe, the twin goals of improving health and reducing health disparities underpinned the US *Healthy People 2010* programme; similarly, New Zealand's health strategy sought 'to reduce inequalities and improve health status' (National Center for Health Statistics, 2001; King, 2000: 3).

In the reports and blueprints which marked the launch of the new health policies, the twin goals of improving health and promoting health equity were

---

**Box 7.4**

'The main influences on health . . . can be thought of as a series of layers, one on top of the other. Overall, there is the major structural environment. Then there are the material and social conditions in which people live and work, determined by various sectors such as housing, education, health care, agriculture and so on. Mutual support from family, friends, neighbours and the local community comes next. Finally, there are actions taken by individuals, such as the food they choose to eat, their smoking and drinking habits. The age, sex and genetic make-up of each individual also play a part, of course, but these are fixed factors over which we have little control.' (Dahlgren and Whitehead, 1991: 11)

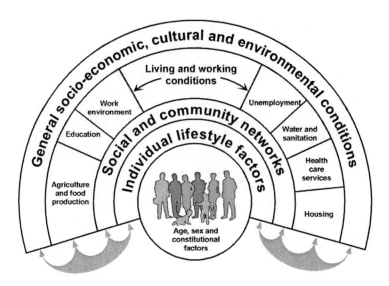

**Figure 7.1**   The main determinants of health

*Source:* reproduced with permission from Dahlgren, G. and Whitehead, M. (1993) 'Tackling inequalities in health: what can we learn from what has been tried?' Working paper prepared for the King's Fund International Seminar on *Tackling Inequalities in Health*, September 1993, Ditchley Park, Oxfordshire (London: King's Fund [mimeo])

typically brought together through an overarching emphasis on tackling determinants (Box 7.5). In the WHO's European strategy of *HFA*, for example, delivering health improvement and health equity is seen to turn on tackling 'basic determinants' and 'root causes of socioeconomic inequities' (WHO Europe, 1999: 4 and 14). In a similar vein, its supporting documents discussed 'the essential role played by the main determinants of health in the generation and development of socioeconomic inequities' (WHO Europe, 2002: 135). At national level, England's policy documents emphasize that the goals of 'improving the health of everyone and the health of the worst off in particular' are to be achieved by tackling 'the determinants of health' and 'the determinants of health inequalities' (Secretary of State for Health, 1999: viii; DoH, 2002: 22–3). What had been canvassed in the 1970s as a new and radical approach to public health is now the lynchpin of mainstream policy.

## 7.3 Models of the social determinants of health

Dahlgren and Whitehead's model is widely known and widely used within the research and policy community, at both national and international level. But it is not the only framework which researchers have developed to capture the

---

**Box 7.5**

---

Northern Ireland's 'new approach to public health . . . aims to improve the health of our people and to reduce inequalities in health . . . by addressing the wider determinants of health.' (DHSSPS, 2000: 6 and 12)

'The determinants of health are considered as "layers of influence" . . . The most immediate layer of influence on health inequalities consists of behavioural patterns such as smoking, diet and physical activity that can be altered directly by the individual but are often affected by social position, economic resources and the material environment. The next layers of influence reflect these so-called "wider determinants" of health inequalities . . . Finally . . . there are the economic, cultural and environmental conditions present in society as a whole . . .' (DoH, 2002: 22–3).

'[T]he determinants of health [are] "layers of influence" . . . tackling health inequalities will require us to address all of these "layers of influence".' (DoH, 2001: 16)

---

social influences on health. Figure 7.2 gives another illustration, selected from a large and growing list (see, for example, Mackenbach *et al.*, 1994; Diderichsen, 1998; Brunner and Marmot, 1999; Hertzman, 1999; Turrell *et al.*, 1999; Whitehead *et al.*, 2000; WHO Equity Team, 2005). Developed for different purposes and audiences, the frameworks vary in their complexity. But across the differences, there are some important similarities.

First, in line with the 1970s critiques which helped to move the concept of social determinants into the policy domain, the models focus on social rather than biological factors: where they are included, genetic and physiological influences figure well down the causal chain as mediators of the influence of 'upstream' determinants. The models typically give little prominence to health care, and many exclude it altogether. But the pattern is not universal. Reflecting the emphasis in the *HFA* strategy on universal primary health care, Dahlgren and Whitehead include health services as a component of people's living and working conditions (Figure 7.1). Its inclusion is supported by evidence that, while environmental improvements were the primary drivers of mortality decline in high-income countries until the middle decades of the twentieth century, improved access to more effective therapies has played an important role in its continuing fall (see Chapter 5, section 5.4).

Second, the upstream factors are frequently represented as a web of influences which have their origins in the structure of society: in 'general socioeconomic, cultural and environmental conditions' (Figure 7.1) and 'social, cultural and economic characteristics of society' (Figure 7.2). These societal-level factors exert their influence on a set of middle-range determinants,

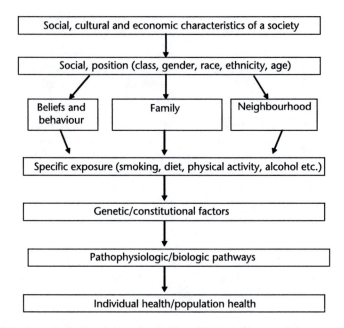

**Figure 7.2** Causal pathways linking the social and biological causes of disease

*Source:* reproduced with permission Najman (2001) 'A general model of social origins of health and wellbeing' in *The Social Origins of Health and Well-being* Eckersley, Dixon and Douglas eds (Cambridge University Press: Cambridge), figure 5.1

labelled 'living and working conditions' and 'social position' in the two models. Health behaviours ('lifestyle factors' and 'specific exposure') are placed further along the causal pathway, and typically as the last of the social influences on health. From this point, genetic and biological factors take over, and are represented as the proximal influences on health.

Figure 7.3 crafts a generic model of the social determinants of health from these two common features. It represents health as the outcome of processes which begin with the *social structure* in which *social position* is embedded. Social position, in turn, mediates access and exposure to a set of *intermediate factors*. These intermediate factors include the social and material environments of home, neighbourhood and workplace, which both provide resources for health and contain risks for health. For example, people's working conditions have been identified as mediating the association between occupation and health. Workers who have limited control over the pace and content of work are at greater increased risk of poor health than those with greater influence over their working conditions (Marmot *et al.*, 1999). Intermediate factors include, too, behaviours which can be either health protecting and enhancing (like exercise) or health damaging (cigarette smoking and energy-dense/

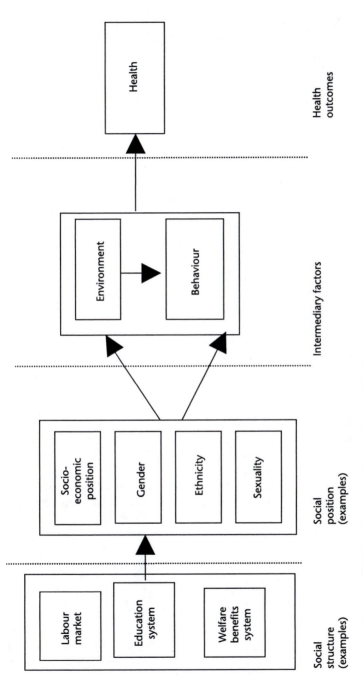

**Figure 7.3** A simplified model of the social determinants of health

nutrient poor diets). Together, the intermediate social factors directly affect our health. Like the models from which it derives, Figure 7.3 signals that intermediate influences have their origins in positional determinants, and positional determinants are inseparable from the broader social structure.

Most models of the social determinants of health conform to this common basic structure. However, the structure is elaborated in different ways. For example, while the typical framework has health (or disease and death) at its endpoint, some models go further. They include societal factors, social positions, specific exposures, health *and* the social consequences of health (see, for example, Mackenbach *et al.*, 1994; Diderichsen *et al.*, 2001; WHO Equity Team, 2005). These frameworks capture the fact that health affects our socioeconomic position and thus our risk of exposure to adverse intermediate factors. In other words, health is both an outcome and a determinant of people's social conditions. Good health makes it easier for people to enter, remain and gain promotion in the labour market, and thus to live and work in low-risk environments. Long-term illnesses and impairments, and the discrimination that can result, makes all this more difficult. Chronic ill health can prevent people entering paid work and can push those in work down the occupational hierarchy and out of the labour market. Thus people with chronic conditions are at a much higher risk of unemployment and poverty, with poor conditions further undermining their health and their independence (Lindholm *et al.*, 2002; Emerson *et al.*, 2005). For individuals, these processes of health-related mobility are clearly critical for their future circumstances, with deteriorating conditions placing their health at further risk. While important for individuals, health-related mobility (or 'health selection' as it is also called) has been found to explain only a small part of the overall socio-economic gradient in health (Blane *et al.*, 1993; Power *et al.*, 1996). As this suggests, the dominant pathway linking social position and health is, as indicated in Figure 7.3, one which runs from social position to health.

As a further elaboration, some models make clear that the social determinants of health are policy sensitive. They 'are influences that are theoretically modifiable by policy' (Dahlgren and Whitehead, 2006: 20). As one example, the model developed by Finn Diderichsen and colleagues includes 'policy' in a box which extends the full length of the causal pathway depicted in Figure 7.3, with arrows indicating that it can impact at all points along it (see Diderichsen, 1998; Whitehead *et al.*, 2001).

Like the models from which it derives, Figure 7.3 is presented as a model of the social determinants of health. But, while not made explicit, inequalities run through all its tiers. This is because, to a greater or lesser extent, inequalities in overarching determinants exist in all societies: in the education system and labour market and in the wider distribution of property and wealth. Unequal structures, in turn, produce inequalities in social positions, with these positional inequalities leaving people unequally exposed to health-damaging environments and behaviours – and therefore unequally at risk of illness, injury and impairment. Figure 7.4 makes this sequential process explicit, signalling that inequalities in structural determinants generate inequalities in positional and intermediate determinants – and thus result in inequalities in health.

As a generic model, Figure 7.4 does not include the elaborations which distinguish some of the frameworks. But, like Figure 7.3, the model could be extended to incorporate the unequal consequences of ill health and impairment. This would be in line with evidence that limiting long-term illness has a greater effect on the circumstances of those who are already disadvantaged. Workers in higher status non-manual jobs have a better chance of staying in employment following the onset of illness than workers in lower status manual work (Bartley and Owen, 1996; Burström *et al.*, 2000). Similarly, Figure 7.4 could explicitly note the role of policy in influencing the cumulative processes – structural, positional and intermediate – which underlie health inequalities by including it as an extra box running under (or over) these social determinants.

Figures 7.3 and 7.4 are highly simplified representations of the pathways linking (unequal) social structures to (unequal) health. A number of schematic aspects need to be highlighted.

First, the determinants – structural, positional, intermediate – are neatly arranged in their own boxes. In reality, their boundaries overlap. As discussed in Chapter 3, social structures and social positions blur at the edges, with many sociologists seeing unequal social positions as constitutive of the unequal structures of which they are part. Similarly, it can be difficult to draw sharp dividing lines between social positions and intermediate factors. People live their socio-economic positions through the conditions with which they are associated. Thus, poor working conditions, poor living conditions and poor neighbourhoods are not separate from disadvantaged social positions: they are its material expression. Sociologists are arguing, too, that consumption patterns, including eating habits and smoking behaviour, are not separate from social class. Instead, they are integral to how people inhabit and display their class position. While policy is typically left outside these boxes, it is also inseparable from the determinants inside them. As the evidence presented in Chapters 5 and 6 indicates, economic and social policy is part of the production of the social structure and social position; it influences, too, the risk factors – both environmental and behavioural – to which populations are exposed.

Second, it is important to remember that models are no more than starting points to understand this social process. The language of fundamental determinants, root causes and causal pathways can convey the impression that health researchers have uncovered a set of iron laws about people's health. This is far from the case. The models signal only that non-clinical factors hold the key to understanding people's health and these factors operate across a range of interconnecting levels, from the macro to the micro.

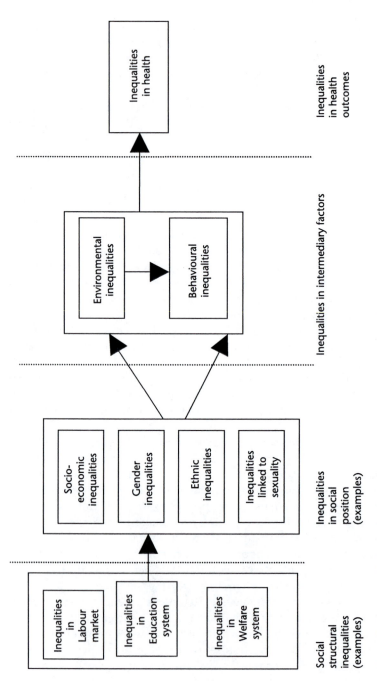

**Figure 7.4** A simplified model of the social determinants of health inequalities

Inequalities in health outcomes

Inequalities in intermediary factors

Inequalities in social position (examples)

Social structural inequalities (examples)

Inequalities in health

Environmental inequalities

Behavioural inequalities

Socio-economic inequalities

Gender inequalities

Ethnic inequalities

Inequalities linked to sexuality

Inequalities in Labour market

Inequalities in Education system

Inequalities in Welfare system

Third, Figures 7.3 and 7.4, like the models from which they derive, provide a cross-sectional snapshot of longitudinal processes. The social structure is not a static monolith. As noted in Chapter 3, it is being produced as children grow up and adults grow older. This temporal perspective is particularly important for understanding the links between social determinants and health outcomes (as Box 7.6 illustrates). This perspective is emphasized in Chapter 10, which discusses how conditions in early life and across the life course have powerful health effects.

## 7.4 Social position as a key determinant of health

In seeking to understand the complex social processes which impact on people's health, researchers have highlighted the centrality of social position. This is because, as Figures 7.3 and 7.4 indicate, it marks the point at which the resources distributed through major social institutions like the labour market enter and shape people's lives. Those occupying advantaged positions in these broader structures therefore 'command most resources (and) are best able to avoid risks, diseases and the consequences of diseases' (Link and Phelan, 1995: 87). In their influential paper, Bruce Link and Jo Phelan argue that it is the association between socio-economic position and differential command over resources which underlie the association between socio-economic position and health. Because socio-economic position continues to mediate access to resources during periods in which societies and major causes of death change, the association between socio-economic position and health persists over time and despite changes in risk factors and killer diseases. For this reason, they accord socio-economic position the status of 'fundamental cause' (see Box 7.7). Fundamental causes of health 'affect multiple disease outcomes through multiple mechanisms and . . . maintain an association with disease even when the intervening mechanisms change' (Link and Phelan, 1995: 80).

---

**Box 7.6**

'[We] need to study exposures at different points in the life course and to recognise that the biological consequences of these exposures may differ depending on when these exposures occur, as well as their duration and intensity. For some diseases, such as heart disease and some forms of cancer, there are exposures of 20 years or more before the health consequences become visible. With heart disease, assessments of 20-year-olds indicate the initial stages of atherosclerosis, yet the adverse health outcomes of these changes are generally not visible for another 20 or 30 years.' (Najman, 2001: 77–8)

---

**Box 7.7**

'A fundamental cause involves access to resources, resources that can help individuals avoid diseases and their negative consequences through a variety of mechanisms. Thus, even if one effectively modifies intervening mechanisms or eradicates some diseases, an association between a fundamental cause and disease will reemerge. As such, fundamental causes can defy efforts to eliminate their effects when attempts to do so focus solely on the mechanisms that happen to link them to disease in a particular situation.' (Link and Phelan, 1995: 81)

'What makes socioeconomic position such a powerful determinant of health is that it shapes people's experience of, and exposure to, virtually all psycho-social and environmental risk factors for health – past, present, and future – and these in turn operate through a very broad range of physiological mechanisms to influence the incidence and course of virtually all major causes of disease and health'. (House and Williams, 2000: 90)

---

As Link and Phelan's critique makes clear, the category of fundamental cause is not restricted to socio-economic position. It encompasses all social positions which embody unequal access to societal resources and unequal exposure to health risks. Ethnicity, gender and sexuality are all seen to qualify as fundamental causes of people's (unequal) health, representing enduring dimensions of both social and health inequality (Krieger, 2000; Mays *et al.*, 2002).

Perspectives which identify social position as central to the explanation of health inequalities turn the spotlight up as well as down the causal pathway depicted in Figure 7.4. They suggest that identifying the intermediate mechanisms through which socio-economic position affects health is only part of the explanatory task. An understanding of the processes which link the social structure to social position is also required. As Michael Marmot put it, 'we cannot ignore how people got where they are' (1997: 9). Sociological research which has focused on how people got where they are suggests that, like other social positions, socio-economic position is itself socially determined. As Chapter 3 noted, it is fashioned through people's interactions with structures and institutions which order and rank them.

The twin tasks of looking upstream from socio-economic position to the social structure and downstream from socio-economic position to health have been tackled by researchers in different disciplinary fields. The processes through which inequalities in social position are produced and maintained have been investigated by social scientists, and particularly by researchers in the disciplines of sociology and social policy. Meanwhile, social epidemiologists have taken the lead in investigating how systematic differences in people's circumstances are related to systematic differences in their health.

The next three chapters explore some of the themes and findings from these two fields of research.

## 7.5 Conclusions

The chapter has provided a brief overview of the concept of the social determinants of health, and the models which health researchers have developed to explain the social production of health to policy-makers. These models, like the composite models provided in Figures 7.3 and 7.4, are schematic representations. They are simplified cross-sectional 'snapshots' of processes which are complex and longitudinal.

But while providing only a partial picture, the models capture a range of social influences on health. They suggest that these influences originate in the social structure and work through people's social positions, shaping their access to the resources which support good health. As a result, inequalities in socio-economic position are associated with marked and persisting inequalities in their health. Chapters 5 and 6 described how these associations have endured through the economic and epidemiologic transitions which marked the development of today's rich societies – and through the accelerated process of change evident in many low- and middle-income countries.

While central to models of health determinants and analyses of health inequalities, people's unequal social positions have not been the primary focus of health research. Instead, these positions have been taken as the starting point, and attention has been directed to understanding the mechanisms through which they affect people's health. The concern has therefore been with the processes which run between (unequal) social positions and (unequal) health in Figures 7.3 and 7.4, processes explored in Chapter 10. But, however rich and detailed the analyses, they leave out the links which connect social structure to social position. It is to some of these pathways that the book now turns.

# 8    Socio-economic inequalities across generations: occupation and education

## 8.1 Introduction

Chapter 7 introduced the models developed by researchers to make sense of how people's health is shaped by the societies in which they live. While the models differ in detail, they all identify a spectrum of social factors which influence people's health. It is the unequal distribution of these factors – and inequalities in social position in particular – which is seen to underlie inequalities in people's health.

Chapters 8 and 9 explore the distal end of the spectrum, focusing on the links between unequal social structures and unequal social positions. Sociological perspectives suggest that inequalities in social positions are both built into the social structure and are produced by individuals as they move through it (see Chapter 3, sections 3.3 and 3.4). The individual processes can be uncovered through standard research methods, like social surveys and ethnographic studies. But the processes by which structures constrain people's lives are harder to capture through such methods. As a result, the major sources of information provide limited information on the stratifying prac- tices of social institutions. They can therefore paint only a partial picture of the mechanisms through which inequalities in people's positions are reproduced. The chapter draws on these partial sources to shed a little light on the processes involved. As in other chapters, it looks particularly at evidence for the UK. This evidence relies primarily on occupation-based classifications of social class (see Chapter 4, section 4.3).

Chapter 8 explores two core dimensions of socio-economic inequality: occupation and education. Occupational inequalities are central because the vast majority of people in high-income societies rely on wages and wage- related benefits for the incomes they and their families need to survive. Only the wealthiest households receive a significant proportion of their income from other sources, like the stock market (Banks *et al.*, 2003; Mishel *et al.*, 2006). The chapter begins by discussing changes in the occupational structure in high-income societies as a backdrop against which to set its review of occupational and educational inequalities. Section 8.3 investigates whether these changes are making the UK a more open and equal society. To do this, it presents evidence from studies which compare the social class in which children are brought up (measured by father's occupation) with the social class they achieve in adulthood (own occupation).

Young people's educational trajectories, and their educational qualifications in particular, have been identified as the major determinant of their future labour market position. Section 8.4 notes that young people across the class hierarchy are spending longer in full-time education and obtaining higher-level qualifications. However, increased participation and improved attainment have not dented the marked inequalities in young people's educational pathways and achievements. Section 8.5 discusses insights from sociological studies which suggest that inequalities have persisted because of the continuing influence of family background, with families providing children with differential access to the resources needed to do well at school and university.

## 8.2 Changes in the labour market

The labour market is widely regarded as the lynchpin of the socio-economic structure (see Chapter 3, section 3.2). In high-income societies, the labour market has undergone a sequence of changes. Economies supported by farming and farming-related occupations have given way to economies based on mining and manufacturing, and more recently to post-industrial economies in which the service sector becomes an increasingly important source of paid work and national wealth. In the countries of northern Europe, as in Canada and the USA, 75 per cent of the labour force is employed in this sector (UNECE, 2004). The service sector covers highly skilled and well-paid jobs in the professions – in law, medicine and accountancy, for example – as well as in business and financial services and in information and communication technologies. The retail, hospitality and leisure industries are also part of the service sector. Shop work, like work in restaurants, call centres, leisure centres and care homes, is lower skilled and much lower paid.

The economic transitions – from agrarian to industrial to post-industrial – which have underpinned the wealth of high-income societies have produced similar occupational structures and labour markets. For example, a shift from manual to non-manual work and an increase in women's employment have been common trends. However, there are also important national differences. In some countries – and the UK and the USA are prime examples – labour markets have become increasingly polarized and incomes increasingly unequal. The section briefly reviews UK experience with respect to these similar and diverging trends.

Through most of the twentieth century, it was manual work which kept the economies of high-income societies going. Thus in the UK until the 1970s, over two-thirds of men with a current or previous job recorded their occupation as manual, with similar proportions found in other rich societies (Fritzell and Lundberg, 2006). Even among women where manual work has traditionally been a less important source of employment, one in two were manual workers (Reid, 1977). Manual work for men was predominantly skilled; women manual workers were concentrated in semi-skilled and unskilled occupations. Since the 1970s, there has been a rapid contraction of the manual sector. As Figure 8.1 suggests, the proportion of men employed in skilled manual work, like that of women in semi-skilled and unskilled manual work, has declined markedly. The compensatory shift towards non-manual work has been most marked at the top of the socio-economic hierarchy. Between 1975 and 2000, the proportion of men in professional and managerial occupations rose by a third, reaching nearly 30 per cent by 2000. Among women, there has been a threefold increase in the proportion employed in these 'top jobs', with the proportion standing at 15 per cent in 2000.

High-income countries have also seen increasing rates of female employment (Morris, 1990; Ruspini and Dale, 2002; Jacobs and Gerson, 2004). Figure 8.2 illustrates this trend in the UK from the early 1970s to the early 1990s by mapping the proportion of young men and women in non-manual service work (managerial, professional and ancillary occupations), in manual work and who are economically inactive. As it suggests, these decades saw a rapid fall in the proportion of young men in manual jobs and of young women who were economically inactive. In consequence, the economic profiles of men and women became increasingly similar. However, this convergence masks their diverging patterns of full-time and part-time work. As in other high-income countries, family life in the UK continues to be resourced by women's unpaid work and by women's investment in child care in particular (Ruspini and Dale, 2002; Jacobs and Gerson, 2004). Becoming a parent has little economic impact on British men: for women, however, it typically means leaving the labour market, to subsequently re-enter into part-time work, lower rates of pay and poorer promotion prospects (Joshi, 2002; Manning, 2006). Thus in the UK, nine in ten fathers with dependent children work full time; among single and cohabiting mothers, the proportion is less than three in ten (Walling, 2005).

Changes in the occupational structure and increasing labour market participation by women are trends found across high-income societies. But other trends have been more strongly evident in the UK than elsewhere. Like the USA, the UK labour market has polarized and the income distribution has become increasingly skewed towards the richest households.

The decline in manual employment has hit working-class families and communities particularly hard (Green, 1999). At the same time, the service

Men

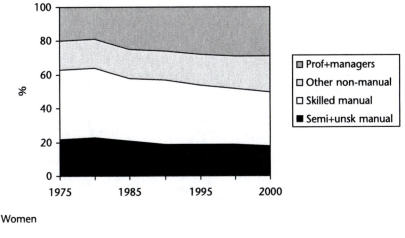

Women

**Figure 8.1** Socio-economic group based on own current or last job, men and women aged 16 and over, 1975 to 2000, Britain

*Note:* Socio-economic group is based on informant's own job or last job if not in employment. Excludes those who have never worked and those in the armed forces

*Source:* ONS, 2001, table 3.14

sector has generated skilled non-manual jobs which are largely inaccessible to those displaced from manual work. With 70 per cent of jobs in Britain restricted to those with educational qualifications, young people who leave school without qualifications can face a life time of moving between low-paid work and unemployment (Green and Owen, 1998; Charlesworth, 2000; Fergusson, 2004). Unemployed workers who manage to get into the labour market typically do so through low-paid work, work which brings a much

Men

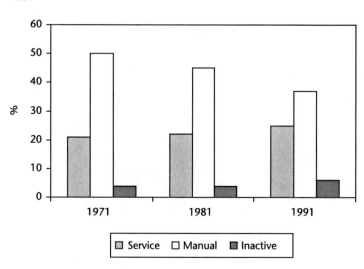

Women

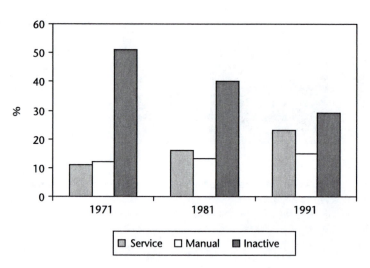

**Figure 8.2** Employment circumstances of young men and women (23 to 27 years) 1971–91, UK

*Source:* adapted from Egerton and Savage 2000, table 1

greater risk of unemployment than higher-paid jobs. Those who remain in work can anticipate little improvement in their relative position: for workers at the bottom of the earnings distribution, wage rises have not kept pace with the rising salary levels of workers in better-paid jobs (Dickens, 2000). As a series of UK studies have noted, the earnings of the already well paid have been increasing much more rapidly than those lower down the wage distribution. The result is a marked widening of inequalities in earnings (T. Atkinson, 2002b). Similar patterns are evident in the USA, with the highest earners doing much better than other workers in the past three decades – and doing particularly well since the mid-1990s (Mishel *et al.*, 2006). But the pattern is not universal: other high-income countries have not seen a similar rise in earnings at the top (Atkinson, 1999).

Changes in the structure of the UK labour market have fuelled a redistribution of paid work and earnings between households (Box 8.1). From the 1970s to 1990s, there was a shift away from households with a single male breadwinner, and a corresponding increase in two-earner and no-earner households (Gregg and Wadsworth, 1996; Atkinson, 1999). Because high earners tend to live with other high earners and no-earner households are concentrated among those with poor job prospects, the trend has contributed to a wider redistribution of income between households.

In the UK, most of the twentieth century saw a narrowing of income inequalities (Atkinson, 1999). From 1900 to 1980, the rich and the 'super-rich' (the top 1 per cent of the income distribution) saw their share of national income shrink (Atkinson, 1999, 2005). But then the equalization of income went into sudden reverse. Inequalities in household income widened sharply. Behind the trend was rapid income growth among those who were already rich while the real incomes of the poorest groups changed little (Goodman and Shepherd, 2002). As a result, households in the top income groups have been taking an increasing proportion of total income. Estimates suggest that the proportion going to the super-rich has climbed from under 6 per cent in the late 1970s to 13 per cent in 2000 (Atkinson, 2005). A similar pattern is evident in the USA. From the 1950s, national income has become increasingly concentrated in the hands of the wealthy. The trend accelerated from the

---

**Box 8.1**

'A century ago, earnings may have come from a male breadwinner and from grown-up children living at home. Today we are more likely to find two-earner couples . . . We also find today a large number of households with zero earned incomes, where all household members are retired, unemployed, sick or otherwise not in the labour force.' (Atkinson, 1999: 57)

1970s, with the real incomes of richer groups rising at a much faster rate than those of the poor (Atkinson, 1999; Mishel *et al.*, 2006).

Some economists see changes in the global economy as explaining the widening differentials in earnings and incomes in the UK and the USA. It is suggested, for example, that the rapidly growing Asian economies have sapped demand for low-skilled labour in high-income countries, pushing up rates of unemployment among low-skilled workers and pushing down their rates of pay. However, this analysis has been challenged. Critics have noted that widening labour market inequalities in the UK and US have not been driven primarily by the changing position of low-paid workers. It is the position of those in the top jobs and the richest households which has changed (Atkinson, 1999, 2002; Glyn, 2006; Mishel *et al.*, 2006). They have noted, too, that the trends which have marked out the UK and the USA over the past 30 years are less evident in other high-income countries. In France, for example, the proportion of total earnings going to the top 1 per cent of earners has remained low and changed little from the 1970s (Glyn, 2006). The broad consensus is therefore that the primary drivers of widening inequalities in earnings and incomes lie in the domestic rather than global arena. In particular, they are the outcome of a sharp change in government policy.

From the late 1970s, governments in the UK and the USA introduced monetarist policies with the aim of deregulating the labour market and reducing public expenditure. Policies progressively restricted the power of trade unions (called labour unions in the USA) to negotiate wages and conditions for manual workers, and weakened frameworks governing minimum wages for low-paid groups (Goodman and Shepherd, 2002; Glyn, 2006; Mishel *et al.*, 2006). At the same time, fiscal and welfare policies in both countries reduced the redistributive impact of tax and welfare benefits. The combined effect of these policies was a rapid widening of income inequalities (Brewer *et al.*, 2006; Mishel *et al.*, 2006). Since 2000, UK policies governing low pay, tax and welfare benefits have combined to reduce inequalities in household income to a modest extent. But by 2005, income inequalities were still higher than they were in 1990 – and much higher than they had been in the 1970s (Brewer *et al.*, 2006). In the USA, policies have continued to be associated with widening inequalities in income and wealth (Glyn, 2006; Mishel *et al.*, 2006). As the examples of the USA and the UK suggest, increasing inequalities in earnings and income are 'to a considerable extent attributable to the reduced redistributive ambitions of the government' (Atkinson, 1999: 286).

Changes in the labour market and the distribution of earnings and incomes provide a backdrop against which to set the persistence of socio-economic inequality across generations. Some processes underlying this persistence are discussed in the sections which follow.

## 8.3 Class origins and class destinations: inequalities across generations

The trend towards non-manual work has had generational effects, with rates of manual work much higher among older workers than among their children. It is a pattern captured in Figure 8.3. Based on a sample of families tracked through the UK Census, the study uses responses to the question on ethnicity in the 1991 Census to place respondents into broad ethnic groups. It includes information for white migrants (parents born outside the UK), white non-migrants (parents born in the UK) and three broad minority ethnic groups (Platt, 2005). Figure 8.3 compares the social class of parents when children were growing up (social class of origin) with the social class which they had achieved by early adulthood (social class of destination). Social class was classified into three categories (professional and managerial, intermediate and routine and manual) in line with the simplified NS-SEC schema (see Chapter 4, section 4.3). It was based on the higher social class of either parent in childhood and, for young people in cohabiting relationships, of either partner in adulthood.

As Figure 8.3 suggests, routine and manual work was the predominant source of parental employment (social class of origin), a pattern found across all ethnic groups. In contrast, it provides the livelihood and defines the class position of only a minority of the younger generation. With the exception of Pakistanis, around half of the younger generation was in a professional or managerial occupation in adulthood (social class of destination).

Within this broad pattern, Lucinda Platt's analysis indicates that social class of origin is more heavily skewed to the routine and manual group for migrant groups than for the white settled population. But the class profile of their children when they reach adulthood is much more similar to the white settled community, with children in the highest social class (professional and managerial) making up the largest category across all ethnic groups. The pattern is consistent with evidence that migration to Britain is associated with downward mobility: newly arrived workers, particularly those facing racial discrimination, take jobs below their educational and occupational levels (Heath and Ridge, 1983). Where the migrant generation experience enforced downward mobility, latent class positions tend to be reasserted through their children, who go on to achieve higher class positions than their parents. In line with this pattern, children from Caribbean, Indian, Black African and white migrant families all had a higher probability of securing a professional or managerial job than their class origins would predict. However, this was not true for Pakistanis and Bangladeshis (Platt, 2005).

For most ethnic groups, Figure 8.3 creates the impression of an upwardly mobile society, with children achieving higher socio-economic positions than

Social class of origin

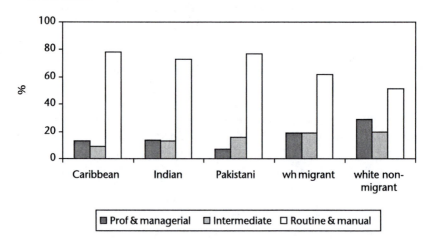

Social class of destination

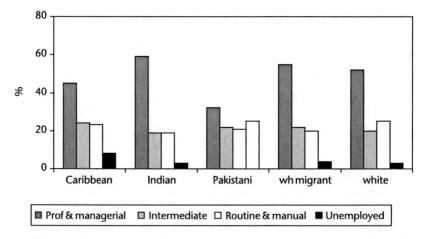

**Figure 8.3** Social class origins and destinations of adults by ethnic group, England and Wales, 2001

*Source:* adapted from Platt, 2005, tables 2.6–2.10

their parents. But, as Figure 8.1 makes clear, these patterns are occurring against a backdrop of major changes in the structure of the labour market. With manual work in rapid decline, the children of manual workers cannot follow in their parent's footsteps: the textile factories, car manufacturing plants and coal mines in which their parents worked have closed. Conversely, a larger pool of non-manual jobs makes it easier for young people from poorer backgrounds to move into a higher social class – and for those born into these more advantaged positions to hold on to them. On its own therefore, the information on class of origin and destination provided in Figure 8.3 cannot tell us whether structural change or individual mobility underlies the divergent class profiles of parents and children.

The challenge is therefore to measure inter generational class positions independent of wider structural changes. The term 'social fluidity' is often used to describe social mobility net of these changes. A widely used approach is to measure the chances of children born into different social classes gaining entry to a particular social class in adulthood: for example, the chances of a child of an unskilled manual worker finding his or her way into the highest occupational social class compared to a child born to parents in this class. A society where there is equality of access to all places in the class structure – in Sen's terms, equal substantive freedom to achieve – is one where the socio-economic position of parents has no effect on the career paths of children. An unequal society would therefore be one where class origins predict class destinations: where the odds of securing a 'top job' are stacked in favour of children from privileged backgrounds and against children from poorer backgrounds.

A long and influential tradition of sociological research has used this approach to study changes and continuities in people's class position across generations. This work has had a strong gender and ethnic orientation, with the focus on fathers and sons in studies in which most respondents are white. As critics have repeatedly pointed out, such studies provide a limited platform on which to build understandings of the patterning of socio-economic inequality in the population as a whole (see, for example, Bottero, 2005; Loury *et al.*, 2005). Nonetheless, these analyses contain an important message: even among white men, there is little evidence of a wide-scale trend towards greater equality.

What emerges, instead, are the generational continuities in class positions. Across high-income societies, it is children born to unskilled manual workers who are most likely to enter unskilled manual occupations, while the chances of entering a professional occupation are highest for those with professional parents (Breen and Rottman, 1995; Breen, 2004). Studies with comparable data on men and women suggest that, while sex segregation in the labour market results in different occupational profiles for men and women, the association between childhood origins and adult destinations is as strong for women as it is for men (Marshall *et al.*, 1997; Breen and Goldthorpe, 2001). Across most of the last century, the strength of this association appears to have changed little in Britain (Marshall *et al.*, 1997; Erikson and Goldthorpe, 2002). Since the 1980s however, there is evidence that Britain has become less socially mobile, with family background having a greater impact on future socio-economic circumstances for children born in the 1970s than those born in the 1950s (Blanden *et al.*, 2001). The country appears to have become more like the USA and less like its neighbours in northern Europe – in the Nordic countries and Germany, for example – where levels of social mobility are higher (Ringdal, 2004; Blanden *et al.*, 2005; Glyn, 2006).

However, while the strength of association between class origins and class destinations varies between countries, it remains significant in all of them (Breen, 2004). What requires explanation is therefore inter genera-tional *im*mobility (Goldthorpe and Mills, 2004). Education is central to the explanation.

## 8.4 Class inequalities in educational trajectories

Changes in the labour markets of high-income societies have been associated with changes in their education systems. Governments have sought to raise educational levels across the population, equipping more young people with the non-manual skills sought by employers. These reforms have been intro-duced against the background of marked social class differences in educational trajectories.

In Britain, for example, secondary education in the 1940s was neither free nor universal. Over 80 per cent of young people left school by 14 and second-ary schools were places where children from advantaged backgrounds gained the qualifications they needed to follow their parents into higher non-manual jobs. Over 60 per cent of children from social class I stayed at school beyond the statutory leaving age; among unskilled manual groups (social class V), the proportion was less than 2 per cent (Douglas and Blomfield, 1958). Not surprisingly, the majority of children from manual backgrounds left school without secondary school level qualifications and did not go on to post-school education: Figure 8.4 captures this pattern for children born in 1940–1. These marked class gradients meant that universities, and the degrees they awarded, belonged almost exclusively to the children of parents in non-manual occupa-tions. Thus, as Figure 8.4 indicates, among children growing up in families where the father was in a professional occupation, one in three had gained entry to a full-time degree course. Among the children of semi-skilled and unskilled workers, the proportion was one in 100.

The late 1940s saw major changes in secondary education in Britain. Universal secondary education was established, with the payment of fees in secondary schools abolished and the statutory leaving age raised from 14 to 15 years. Since then, further large-scale reforms have been introduced, including the introduction of non-selective secondary schools (comprehensive schools) open to children across the ability range. In addition, the statutory leav-ing age has been raised to 16 years, a new integrated system of secondary

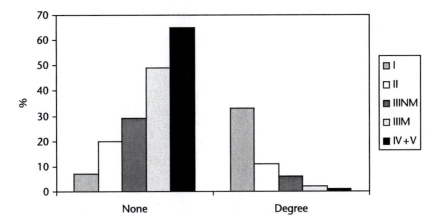

**Figure 8.4** Highest level of education attained by children born 1940–1 by social class of father, Britain

*Note:* 'None' indicates no passes at O levels or Scottish Leaving Certificates and no post-school course

*Source:* adapted from Reid, 1977, table 6.17

---

**Box 8.2**

- In the 1960s, over 60 per cent of 15-year-olds had left school; today, 70 per cent of 16-year-olds are still in full-time education (Reid, 1977; DfES, 2003).
- In the early 1970s, 5 per cent of men and 2 per cent of women had a degree; in the early 2000s, the proportions are 15 per cent and 16 per cent. Among 25 to 34-year-olds, 25 per cent of men and 23 per cent of women now have a degree (Reid, 1977; ONS, 2004).

---

examinations has been established to enable more children to gain qualifications, and higher education has undergone major expansion. Examples of the effects of these changes are given in Box 8.2. As it suggests, mass full-time education no longer ends at age 14 but increasingly extends to the late teenage years and beyond.

Longer years of study are associated with a more educated population. In every social class, the proportion staying on at school and gaining educational qualifications has risen (Marshall *et al.*, 1997; DfES, 2003). But inequalities in educational attainment remain pronounced. Figure 8.5 captures these inequalities in England and Wales for the key benchmark of achievement at secondary school level: having a General Certificate of Secondary Education (GCSE) in five or more subjects at grade A* to C. Family social class is assigned on the basis of parental occupation using the Registrar General's schema; in

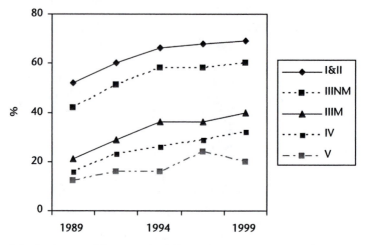

**Figure 8.5** Attainment of five or more GCSE grades A* to C at age 16 by parental social class, England and Wales, 2002

*Source:* adapted DfES 2003, table A

two-parent households, the occupation with the higher status is used. Figure 8.5 suggests that wide inequalities in educational attainment characterized the 1990s, and that the gap increased between children with parents in professional and managerial occupations (social class I and II) and in unskilled manual occupations (social class V). Trends from 2000 point to no narrowing of the attainment gap (DfES, 2003).

Like the UK, other high-income societies have seen a major expansion of post-school education. This expansion has increased the chances of all young people getting qualifications and gaining higher-level qualifications. However, because qualifications provide the gateway into higher education and vocational training, it has favoured those who are already doing well from the educational system (Gangl *et al.*, 2004). These young people are disproportionately drawn from advantaged backgrounds. Thus from 1900 to 1970, UK studies uncovered 'a widening gap between the social classes in terms of the proportion completing higher-tertiary education' (Marshall *et al.*, 1997: 113). From the 1970s, 'the expansion of higher education in the UK has benefited those from richer backgrounds far more than poorer people' (Blanden *et al.*, 2005: 12). Figure 8.6 captures this trend. It shows the higher education participation rates of young people in the late 1970s, late 1980s and late 1990s (Machin, 2003). Across these decades, participation rates among those from the richest families increased steadily, from 27 per cent to 46 per cent; among those in the lowest income quintile, the proportion rose from 9 per cent to 15 per cent.

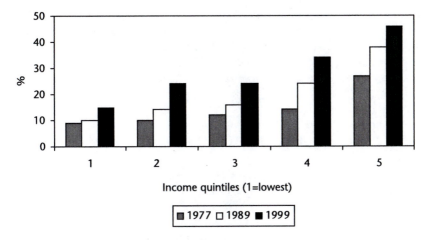

**Figure 8.6** Higher education participation among 19-year-olds by parental income (quintiles) in the late 1970s, 1980s and 1990s

*Source:* Machin, 2003, table 2

Educational inequalities, evident both in the past (Figure 8.4) and present (Figures 8.5 and 8.6), play a powerful role in maintaining class inequalities across generations. This is because class origins influence educational trajectories, and educational trajectories influence class destinations. It is how well young people do, not how long they study, which appears to matter most: the evidence from mobility studies suggests that inequalities in educational qualifications, rather than in years of education, are driving inequalities in adult social class (Marshall *et al.*, 1997).

But education is not only a mechanism of social *im*mobility. Because educational qualifications help secure socio-economic advantage in adulthood, doing well at school and university provides a ladder up the class structure for children from more disadvantaged backgrounds. Thus among young people from poorer families who go on to higher education, the majority progress to jobs unobtainable without the qualifications it provides (Brennan and Shah, 2003; Elias and Purcell, 2004). In the study on which Figure 8.3 is based, educational qualifications were found to explain why the children of migrant groups – Caribbeans, Black Africans, Indians and Chinese as well as white migrants – had a greater chance of entering social class I in adulthood than comparable white non-migrants (Platt, 2005). It is a finding which points to the strong academic-orientation of minority ethnic groups, and one maintained in the face of economic disadvantage and racial discrimination (Modood, 2004; see also Chapter 3, section 3.4). As qualitative studies suggest, parents place great value on education for their children (Archer and Francis, 2006; Barn, 2006). It is a point underlined by the Caribbean mother quoted in

Box 8.3. But educational qualifications do not appear to work as effectively for Bangladeshi and Pakistani children. Platt's analysis suggests that ethnicity is a marker for a range of economic inequalities and cultural differences which may be combining to make education a less effective route into professional and managerial occupations for Bangladeshi and Pakistani young people (Platt, 2005).

## 8.5 Class inequalities in educational opportunities

If, as sociologists suggest, inequalities in educational attainment lie behind occupational inequalities, what drives inequalities in educational attainment? The broad answer is that educational inequalities are the outcome of inequalities in the environments which parents are able to provide for their children, inequalities which the education system appears to compound rather than compensate for. The biological effects of these environmental inequalities, which operate from conception, through infancy and into adolescence, are explored in Chapter 10; here the focus is on some of the social processes.

Bourdieu's concept of cultural capital was introduced in Chapter 3, section 3.4. He developed it to help make sense of 'the unequal scholastic achievement of children originating from different social classes' (1986: 243). Unequal achievement, he argued, resulted from an educational system that demanded, tested and rewarded competences which are class-based and class specific: competences that children from advantaged backgrounds acquire and practise routinely in the process of growing up. Parents who can take their advantages for granted – their career, their high and steady income, their home, their health – can invest money and energy in their children's development. Studies suggest they deploy their privileged resources to actively manipulate their children's environment, engaging in what has been evocatively described as the 'concerted cultivation' of their children (Lareau, 2003). Annette Lareau's US study uncovered patterns noted in the UK (see, for example, Reay, 1998). She found that middle-class parents fed their children 'a

---

**Box 8.3**

'Young people need education in school. Without education you get nowhere in life. That's the main point. I always say to my kids, "When you go to school, it's for you to learn and not mess about, because when it comes for you to leave school and you've got no education, it doesn't matter if the teachers don't like you, she's not there to be liked, she's there to teach." I always tell them that. Without education, you get nowhere in life.' (Mother quoted in Barn, 2006: 54)

steady diet of adult-organized activities' (Lareau, 2003: 3). They meticulously planned their children's lives, organizing how and with whom they spent their time. As the British mother quoted in Box 8.4 suggests, childhood is a tightly regulated sequence of educational activities, with the school day followed by an intensive out-of-school programme. In contrast, the lives of the poorer parents in Lareau's study were more likely to be dominated by economic insecurity and material shortages, experiences which brought a different perspective on parenthood. Crucial responsibilities were to keep the family going and to prepare their children for the hard knocks that life would bring. Parents therefore placed more value on child-organized activities than parent-organized ones. They emphasized the importance of children developing skills to negotiate, survive and thrive in risky environments, working out as they did so how and with whom they spent their time.

These different styles of parenting nurture different sets of competences in children, each adapted to its environment and held in high regard within its cultural setting. However, the competences which matter at school and in the workplace are the ones more easily produced in middle-class homes. Children who have been concertedly cultivated by their parents therefore arrive at school expecting that their teachers will, metaphorically and literally, 'speak their language'. There is a cultural congruence between home and school, what Bourdieu would call a shared habitus (see Chapter 3, section 3.4 for a discussion of this concept). Once inside the school gates, further advantages await them. Embodying the cultural capital valued by the education system, they can expect to receive more positive attention than children who teachers find less rewarding to teach (Box 8.5).

Children from middle-class homes also have parents who can help to smooth their way through the education system. As Diane Reay's studies suggest, middle-class parents can successfully navigate the school system on

---

**Box 8.4**

'Our children strike a good balance between school, extra-curricular stuff, being with their friends and having downtime. Our oldest boy, Jack, who's 12, does cricket, football, guitar lessons, basketball and extra maths tuition. Rosie, who's nine, has choir followed by Brownies on Monday, swimming every Friday, trampolining on Sunday mornings and maths class with Jack every Tuesday after her netball . . . In some families we know, the kids do something after school virtually every day of the week . . . There's definitely a social premium put on your kids doing extra stuff. You do compare what you are doing with neighbours and friends. If Jack and Rosie weren't doing "enough" extra-curricular things I'd feel I wasn't a good enough mum.' (Campbell, 2006: 3)

---

**Box 8.5**

---

'There is evidence that teachers develop preferences for certain students who are perceived as college bound and motivated, generally children from privileged families. Children from disadvantaged families, in contrast, are given less positive attention, fewer learning opportunities, and less reinforcement for instances of good performances. Students, in turn, are influenced by their teachers' feelings about their abilities, and it has been shown that teacher expectations about their students' achievements influence not only teacher–student interactions but student performance.' (Schoon *et al.*, 2004: 387)

---

behalf of their children, thus ensuring a quality of education unavailable to many poorer children (see Chapter 3, section 3.4). As these advantaged young people move onto secondary education, most will expect to stay beyond the statutory leaving age and go on to university (Burchardt, 2005). Parents often help them financially in realizing these goals. Students from middle-class backgrounds receive more financial support in the form of parental gifts and long-term loans than those from poorer backgrounds, enabling them to leave home to go to higher-prestige universities and to graduate with less debt (Callender and Wilkinson, 2004; Furlong and Cartmel, 2005).

In contrast, and not surprisingly, children from poorer backgrounds can experience a sense of dislocation and estrangement at every stage of their journey through the education system. By the time children from manual groups reach adolescence, the majority intend to leave school when legally permitted to do (at 16 in the UK) and very few expect to go to university (Burchardt, 2005). Those who do are more likely to apply for and enrol on vocational courses at local universities, seeking to reduce costs and to stay close to their cultural roots (Box 8.6). Studies have recorded, too, how black young people, both middle and working class, may prefer local universities in black and urban areas in preference to more prestigious universities which are (inevitably) white and middle class (Box 8.7).

While education has been identified as the critical link between social class of origin and social class of destination, it is not the whole story. A consistent finding is that children's social backgrounds influence their future careers independently of their educational qualifications. In other words, class origins influence class destinations over and above their effect on educational attainment. Thus, even when measures of ability and effort are included in the analysis, children's social origins affect their social destinations (Savage, 2000; Breen and Goldthorpe, 2001). Children from working-class backgrounds 'need to show substantially more merit than children from more advantaged class origins in order to enter similarly desirable

---

**Box 8.6**

'They [disadvantaged young people] often chose courses at institutions closest to their parents' home so as to limit costs; where it could be avoided, young people did not leave home and sometimes chose courses on the basis of the lowest daily bus fares . . . In colleges and universities, economic and cultural barriers impacted on experiences. Less advantaged students tended to follow more complex and protracted pathways through education, were more likely to drop out or to forgo the opportunity to fulfil their academic potential. The fear of debt affected many decisions while both economically and culturally they found it difficult to integrate within peer groups dominated by the middle classes.' (Furlong and Cartmel, 2005: 1–2)

---

**Box 8.7**

'I was put off Goldsmiths' [a university in London], the interview was really, really stressful. It was like what I'd imagined to be a conversation round a dinner table in a really upper-class, middle-class family and I was like "Oh my God, I'm not ready for this. This is not me". It was awful' (Maggie, white English working-class further education student, quoted in Reay, 2005: 922)

'I was offered two university places at East London University and Lancaster to study mechanical engineering. At first I wanted to go to Lancaster, it has one of the best reputations for the course. What put me off was the place itself. I didn't see a black face. At the Open Day I'm the only black person. I kept thinking "where are all the black people" . . . It was a really white place and I didn't think I belonged . . . I thought to myself "I can't live here for 4 years. It's too white". I wouldn't be able to settle down and that would affect my work. I'd always be running back to London or Leeds, just to see some black faces and feel comfortable. So I decided London was the place for me.' (David, age 21, quoted in Reynolds, 2006: 277)

---

class positions in the course of their adult lives' (Breen and Goldthorpe, 2001: 82). This suggests that class inequality operates outside as well as through the education system. There is evidence that it increasingly does so. In recent decades, the effect of educational attainment on class destination has grown weaker, both in the UK and in other high-income countries (Marshall *et al.*, 1997; Breen, 2004). In today's advanced economies, it appears that educational attainment is becoming a less important mechanism through which class inequality is maintained. The transmission of cultural capital appears to play an increasingly important role in the persistence of advantage across generations (Box 8.8).

---

**Box 8.8**

'In modern economies . . . increasing economic value now attaches to individual attributes of a kind less likely to be achieved through the educational system than ascribed through processes of socialisation within more generally advantaged families and communities . . . Men and women with advantaged class backgrounds acquire, more or less as a matter of course, attributes which help them maintain their position even if their educational attainments are only modest.' (Erikson and Goldthorpe, 2002: 40)

'There is a growing literature which suggests that social skills, personality traits, and cultural resources may be as important as educational certificates in hiring and promotion decisions or, more broadly, in determining who gets ahead'. (Esping-Andersen, 2004: 298)

---

## 8.6 Conclusions

The chapter has focused on education and occupation as two key constituents of socio-economic inequality. The key data sources focus on individuals rather than social structures, with the result that more is known about the processes at the individual rather than institutional level.

The chapter noted that occupations which rely on the inheritance of property – farms, small holdings and small businesses – have been in long-term decline. Conversely, occupations which are not in the gift of parents to bequeath to their children, like those in the service sector, have been increasing. Such changes might be expected to open up societies, giving children from poorer backgrounds a greater chance of getting to the top. Studies of social mobility provide little evidence that this is the case. Once changes in the occupational structure are taken into account, children's social origins continue to exert a powerful influence on their social destinations. In the UK, the association between the socio-economic position of parents and children appears to be increasing rather than weakening.

Educational trajectories have been identified as the major route through which privilege is passed down the generations. This means that social background influences social prospects indirectly, with parents in higher socio-economic positions securing future advantages for their children by helping them gain educational qualifications (Glass, 1954). Across high-income societies, young people who attain higher levels of qualifications have a higher chance of accessing professional and secure jobs, while those with lower or no qualifications are more likely to be restricted to low-skilled and temporary jobs. The evidence suggests, too, that changes in the labour market and the education systems have done little to break this pattern. Instead, analyses suggest that it is young people from more advantaged backgrounds and with higher educational levels who are benefiting most from the expansion of educational opportunities and the upgrading of the occupational structure found across high-income societies (Gangl *et al.*, 2004; Breen and Rottman, 1995). But education is not the only route through which unequal starting places anticipate unequal destinations. Chapter 9 turns to another set of pathways through which class inequalities are maintained.

# 9 Socio-economic inequalities across people's lives: partnership and parenthood

## 9.1 Introduction

The previous chapter noted how inequalities in people's socio-economic circumstances have persisted over time and across generations. In the UK, they show little sign of diminishing; instead, class origins appear to have an increasing effect on class destinations. Chapter 8 discussed the role of education in the continuities in class position from childhood to adulthood. Such evidence suggests that inequalities are sustained by a single and linear trajectory, running from the socio-economic environment of the natal family through the education system to the labour market.

These understandings of the persistence of socio-economic inequality are grounded in studies comparing the occupations of fathers and sons in white families. This narrow focus is slowly broadening, with social researchers looking beyond occupation and beyond white men. Analyses which compare the socio-economic circumstances of parents and children in multi-ethnic populations have found, too, that education helps to explain patterns of social mobility and immobility. But children's experiences at school are only one part of a wider process through which advantage and disadvantage is transmitted across the generations. Other routes are involved. In particular, traditional approaches to social mobility obscure how patterns of partnership and parenthood are integral to transmission processes. Thus our childhood circumstances influence our choice of partner and whether, when and in what circumstances we have children – and these aspects of our private lives in turn influence our current and future socio-economic circumstances.

The chapter turns a spotlight on domestic trajectories. The section below presents an overview of these trajectories, noting their particular importance for women's socio-economic circumstances in adulthood – and therefore for the circumstances in which the next generation of children are born and brought up. The chapter then discusses young people's changing pathways into partnership and parenthood, pointing to evidence that young motherhood forms part of a trajectory of longer-term disadvantage. The chapter focuses on the experiences of the small proportion of young women who become mothers before their early twenties. Their accounts suggest that, for many, motherhood is imagined and experienced, not as a pathway to social exclusion, but as a mode of social inclusion. Young motherhood can provide an identity which, as Sen puts it, 'they have reason to value' (1999: 74). Again, the evidence that the chapter presents relates primarily to the UK, but reference is made to wider patterns across high-income societies.

Most of what is known about domestic pathways comes from surveys of individuals. These pathways are embedded in wider social structures, structures which, as earlier chapters have noted, are poorly captured in social surveys. While individual-level data reveal little about the operation of the education system and the labour market, these institutions have ineluctable effects on people's lives. The sections below should therefore be read with an appreciation that, behind the data on individuals, is a network of powerful institutions which unequally resource their lives.

## 9.2 Partnership, parenthood and adult socio-economic position

The economic transitions – from agrarian to industrial and post-industrial – which created today's high-income societies, have been associated with changes in family life. The extended multigenerational households found in agriculture-based societies have given way to smaller nuclear families based on marriage, a family structure which, in turn, is evolving into an increasingly diverse set of household patterns. The different domestic pathways through which young people make their way to adulthood have a place in the story of how socio-economic inequalities are reproduced across generations. Like educational pathways, these pathways are shaped by circumstances in childhood.

Our childhood circumstances influence our choice of partner. Today, as in the past, we tend to form cohabiting partnerships with people who have similar social backgrounds. The process is somewhat quaintly called 'assortative mating'. It means that a privileged start in life not only increases a young person's chances of gaining educational qualifications and entering a professional and managerial occupation; it also makes it more likely that they will settle down with a similarly highly educated and well-paid partner (Ermisch *et al.*, 2006). The result is a new household resourced by the cultural and economic capital of two families of origin, and the incomes of two high-earning adults. Conversely, the new households formed by young adults whose formative years were spent in poverty are likely to be ones in which neither partner has high educational qualifications and high earnings. Focusing on the UK, Box 9.1 provides a glimpse of this process of assortative mating

---

**Box 9.1**

---

The Millennium Cohort Study, a study of 18,800 UK babies born in 2000–1, found a strong association between the socio-economic position of mothers and partners. Among those living with a partner, over two-thirds of mothers whose current or last job was a managerial and professional one had a partner in the same socio-economic group; conversely, nearly half of the mothers who had never worked had a partner in a routine or semi-routine occupation (data from Bradshaw *et al.*, 2005).

---

among today's parents. It is a process which amplifies the effects of widening differentials in educational attainment and earnings on household income outlined in Chapter 8. Because 'like lives with like' inequalities in income are wider than they would otherwise be (Atkinson, 1999). If, instead, the typical pattern was for young people from privileged backgrounds and with high earning power to settle down with partners without these advantages, inequalities in household incomes would be greatly attenuated.

Partnership and parenthood are particularly important influences on women's socio-economic position. Being and remaining married protects women's living standards (Box 9.2). Thus in the UK, single women are more likely to live in low-income households than single men (Women and Equality Unit, 2004). Entry into marriage has a more marked effect on women's employment patterns, earnings and household incomes than on men's (Bartley *et al.*, 2002). Exit from marriage through separation and divorce brings a more rapid and sharper fall in income for women than men (Jarvis and Jenkins, 1998). Divorced women, particularly those in younger age groups, have lower rates of employment than both married women and divorced men (Wertheimer and McRae, 1999; Perry *et al.*, 2000).

Becoming a parent has much higher economic opportunity costs for women than men. In high-income countries like the UK, women and men's employment rates are almost identical (at around 90 per cent) until they become parents (Paull, 2006). Becoming a father makes very little difference to

---

**Box 9.2**

---

'The route to a high lifetime standard of living is different for men and women – for men the labour market is of prime importance whereas for women it remains the marriage market . . . Getting married and staying married is virtually essential for a woman to reach the top part of the [lifetime] income distribution'. (Evandrou and Falkingham, 1995: 182 and 169)

either a man's current or future employment position. Becoming a mother makes a major and lasting difference for a woman. The traditional – and still persisting – gendered division of parental duties means that women take primary responsibility for the care of the first child as well as of children born subsequently (Calderwood *et al.*, 2005; Crompton *et al.*, 2005). The rate of employment among women drops to around 30 per cent in the year after birth and, while it climbs subsequently, remains well below that of men for the rest of their working lives (Paull, 2006).

Gendered patterns of lone parenthood contribute to the unequal economic effects of having children. Women are both more likely to become a lone parent and to devote a larger part of their lives to caring for children alone than men (Rendall *et al.*, 2001). In the UK, lone mothers are at a much higher risk of poverty than mothers in a cohabiting relationship (Bradshaw *et al.*, 2005). Even in countries like Sweden which have invested in universal, high-quality child care and have a more generous system of welfare benefits, lone mothers have lower rates of employment and higher rates of poverty than lone fathers and mothers in two-parent households (Wong *et al.*, 1993).

## 9.3 Widening inequalities in domestic trajectories

The past 50 years have seen major changes in people's domestic lives in high-income societies. In the 1950s and 1960s, the majority of young people made an ordered progression from school to work in their mid to late teens (Gangl *et al.*, 2004). In Britain in the 1960s, two-thirds of young people left school at the minimum leaving age and the majority went straight into full-time employment (Bynner, 1999). Fifty years ago, too, the majority of young people followed a uniform pathway into marriage and parenthood. For example, among women born in Britain in the 1940s, 60 per cent were married by the age of 23. By 23, too, over 50 per cent of women had had their first child (Kiernan and Eldridge, 1987; Ferri and Smith, 2003). While women from more advantaged backgrounds tended to marry and become mothers later than women from manual background families, the normative pattern in all social classes was one of early entry into marriage followed by parenthood by their mid-twenties.

From the 1970s, these normative transitions to adulthood began to change and diversify. The pattern was first evident and has been most pronounced in the early industrializing countries of northern Europe and North America. Labour market changes have been an important part of this process of change (Gangl *et al.*, 2004). In Britain, as in other high-income countries, recent decades have seen the collapse of the manual sectors of the labour market which traditionally provided employment for young people leaving school at the minimum leaving age and with few qualifications (see Chapter 8, section

8.2). Since the 1970s, job opportunities both for semi-skilled and unskilled manual employment (for young women) and for apprenticeships into skilled manual work (for young men) have shrunk (Green, 1999). Governments have responded by investing in youth training programmes and the expansion of post-school education – and young people have chosen (or been constrained) to extend the period of full-time education beyond the minimum leaving age and defer entry into full-time employment (see Chapter 8, section 8.4).

The lengthening of the education-to-work transition has been associated with a lengthening of domestic transitions, with young people delaying entry into cohabitation/marriage and into parenthood. From the 1970s, birth rates to women under the age of 20 fell and birth rates to women in their thirties rose as women increasingly delayed having children. In contrast to the previous generation, the majority of women born in the 1970s were not mothers by their mid-twenties; instead nearly 70 per cent were still childless (Summerfield and Babb, 2004). Recent decades have also seen an increasing proportion of women opting out of motherhood, breaking with the normative assumption that having children is every woman's destiny (Summerfield and Babb, 2004).

Greater diversity in women's reproductive trajectories is matched by greater diversity in the families into which children are born. In many high-income countries – like France, Denmark, Sweden and the USA – marriage is increasingly only one of a range of family structures in which children are growing up (Kiernan, 2004; Summerfield and Babb, 2004). The UK is part of this trend, with the proportion of children born outside marriage increasing from under 10 per cent in 1970 to 40 per cent today (Kiernan, 2004; Bartley *et al.*, 2005). These parenting patterns are strongly related to ethnicity. In Indian, Pakistani and Bangladeshi families, very few children (under 3 per cent in 2000) are born outside marriage. The proportion is appreciably higher among babies born to mothers in other ethnic groups, including white, mixed parentage, Black-African and Black-Caribbean mothers (Bartley *et al.*, 2005).

The trend towards later childbearing and away from marriage is also strongly patterned by socio-economic position. Among the white population, the postponement of parenthood has been particularly marked among women and men from non-manual backgrounds and with educational qualifications. Conversely, it is young people without these advantages who are more likely to become parents by their mid-twenties and outside marriage (Singh *et al.*, 2001; Sigle-Rushton, 2005). Some of the complex patterns involved are captured in Figure 9.1. It is drawn from a contemporary British study of women (Inskip *et al.*, 2006). Figure 9.1 maps the educational and domestic profile of women aged 22 to 34 by their social class of origin (based on father's occupation) using the UK's official socio-economic classification, the NS-SEC (see Chapter 4, section 4.3). As Figure 9.1 indicates, only a minority of women in this age group have no educational qualifications and few have followed the normative pattern of the 1950s and 1960s and become mothers by their early

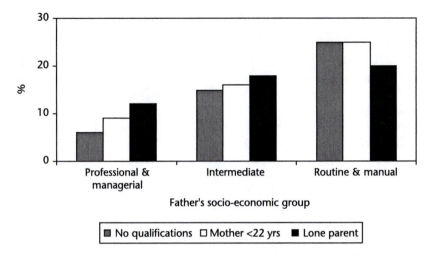

**Figure 9.1**   Educational and domestic trajectories by childhood socio-economic circumstances (father's occupation), women aged 22 to 34, Britain 1998–2002

*Note:* Childhood socio-economic circumstances are based on father's occupation at the time of the woman's birth, categorized using NS-SEC; percentage of lone parents is based on women who were mothers at the time of recruitment to the survey

*Source:* unpublished data reproduced with permission of Southampton Women's Survey

twenties. But marked socio-economic gradients in educational and domestic trajectories remain. These gradients are evident for leaving school without qualifications (with less than five passes at grades A* to C at the standard secondary examination). The proportion having their first baby by the age of 22 is at its lowest among women from the most advantaged class backgrounds (9 per cent) and highest among women from the most disadvantaged backgrounds (25 per cent). Among those who are mothers, the rates of lone parenthood are also highest among women whose fathers were in routine and manual occupations.

Early motherhood is associated with poorer circumstances in later adulthood, effects that remain after account is taken of childhood circumstances (Hobcraft and Kiernan, 2001; Ermisch, 2003). As this suggests, both early-life disadvantage and early motherhood can take a long-term toll on the socio-economic prospects of women and their children. Early parenthood has therefore been identified as a mechanism through which the disadvantages experienced by the current generation of young people merge into disadvantages experienced by the next. As one major review of social exclusion put it, 'teenage motherhood, perhaps more than any other status, epitomizes the problem: early school leaving, no qualifications, poor job or youth training, pregnancy and childbirth, poor prospects of ever getting a decent job, family poverty' (Bynner and Pan, 2002: 25).

It is important to remember, however, that childhood disadvantage does not inevitably lead young women into teenage motherhood. As Figure 9.1 indicates, the majority (75 per cent) of those with parents in manual and routine jobs were not mothers by their early twenties. Further, the depiction of teenage motherhood as epitomizing the problem of social exclusion can be and has been criticized for being implicitly normative: for taking the transitions which exemplify what it is to be young, white and middle class as the yardstick against which alternative trajectories are judged (Burton, 1990; Fergusson, 2004). Judged against this standard, it can be difficult to appreciate that there are young women who, like the majority in the 1950s and 1960s, have different priorities and life plans. While some of their contemporaries may put greater weight on building their future careers, they may feel that investing early in family identities and family relationships provides a more certain and rewarding route into adulthood. The next section turns to qualitative studies for insights into the values affirmed by early motherhood.

## 9.4 Young motherhood

Most of what is known about early parenthood comes from quantitative studies which cast it as a marker of past disadvantage and future risk. There are far fewer studies which record young people's views and experiences. There is, however, a small clutch of qualitative studies of young people's experiences of growing up which shed a tangential light on early parenthood. There is also a larger pool of qualitative studies of young mothers' lives.

In the first category is an ethnographic study by Rachel Thomson. It focused on two contrasting areas in the UK. In the first area, a predominantly white executive commuter belt, young people were transported to school and spent little time together in the public spaces of the street and the shopping centre. Instead, their leisure time was 'highly structured and serviced by parents' (Thomson, 2000: 413). Experiencing little cultural dissonance between home and school, the young people described how respect and popularity could be combined by doing well at school, deferring sexual relationships and rejecting early parenthood. As Thomson points out, for young people destined to do well at school and to progress to university and a well-paid career, 'there is little to be gained from sex and potentially much to lose', particularly for young women (2000: 424).

The second area was an ethnically diverse public housing estate with high rates of unemployment and crime. Young people lived within walking distance of the school and spent their out-of-school time in the same public spaces. Like their more advantaged peers in the leafy suburbs, they recognized the importance of education for future employment. But they knew that respect and popularity were hard to secure through success in examinations.

Over time, those striving to do well at school were forced to abandon their dreams of higher education and a successful career, and adjust instead to the reality of leaving school with minimal qualifications and a future of low-paid and insecure work (Thomson *et al.*, 2003). Not surprisingly, it was a prospect which encouraged many to look beyond the school and the labour market for a positive vision of themselves and their future. They quickly learned that 'young men had much to gain from the cultivation of sexual reputations, and young women had much to gain from the experience and authority of motherhood' (Thomson, 2000: 425). As Box 9.3 suggests, an identity anchored in early motherhood offered opportunities for individual maturation and social status denied by other pathways to adulthood. It also provided a positive alternative to local youth cultures, which young women experienced as dominated by young men cultivating a hard and sexualized masculinity (Thomson, 2000).

Qualitative studies of young mothers' lives pick up the story of the transmission of disadvantage where the ethnographic studies of young people end. A systematic review of UK qualitative studies brings out the common themes which emerge. Across the studies, white and black mothers spoke of the material hardship and social stigma that they faced on a daily basis (McDermott and Graham, 2005). But the mothers spoke, too, of their positive experiences of motherhood and the importance they attached to their relationship with their children (Box 9.3).

The priority that young mothers attached to their maternal identity helped to guide them through often complex relationships with their child's father. The capacity of male partners to provide a home – specifically, to be a supportive partner, engaged father and economic provider – was questioned

---

**Box 9.3**

'It has made me more settled in, like, myself, because I have a goal now and I have something to achieve and I have to bring her up the best way I can and give her the best of everything and do what I can to help her grow up and not be like how I am.' (Young mother quoted in Corlynon and McGuire, 1999: 140)

'I loved being pregnant. I thought it was brilliant . . . had this feeling of being worthy of something and I just felt . . . radiant all the time. And I was looking forward to having the baby . . . I couldn't wait for this little thing to look after and love.' (Young mother quoted in Burghes and Brown, 1995: 50)

'I'm making the best of what I've got and I think I am doing a damn good job. I am proud of the way I handle things.' (Young mother quoted in Mitchell and Green, 2002: 15)

by the young women, with the mother–child dyad seen as a more certain source of intimacy. The mother–child relationship, in turn, formed part of a vertical female kin structure linking the generations (young mother, mother and grandmother). Studies have documented how, in communities where economic opportunities for both men and women are limited, motherhood by one's early twenties and grandmotherhood by one's early forties brings and binds the generations together. As Linda Burton notes in her study of low-income African American families in north-east USA, 'women shorten generations through early childbearing to create what is perceived to be a viable female support system' (1990: 137). Like the families of advantaged young people, families work hard to facilitate their children's pathways into adulthood. Thus the young mothers in the studies spoke of how their relatives, and their mothers in particular, helped to secure the resources needed to care for a young child. Despite their own disadvantaged circumstances, their families worked to provide money, accommodation in the parental home, baby clothes and equipment, and food, as well as child care. The kinship structure also protected young mothers from exposure to the stigma and surveillance they experienced elsewhere (McDermott and Graham, 2005).

Like the quantitative evidence discussed in section 9.2, the evidence from qualitative studies suggests that disadvantage increases the chances, that a young woman will make an accelerated transition to adulthood. But, unlike the quantitative studies, qualitative evidence suggests that young motherhood is not simply, or straightforwardly, a pathway to social exclusion. It can be experienced, instead, as a mode of social inclusion: a gateway into adulthood which opens the door to a valued maternal identity and a support structure which recognizes and affirms it.

## 9.5 Conclusions

Chapters 8 and 9 have focused on inequalities in socio-economic position, inequalities identified by researchers as the underlying cause of health inequalities. The chapters have looked at how inequalities in socio-economic position persist across generations: at how advantaged circumstances in childhood pave the way to advantaged circumstances in adulthood while childhood disadvantage increases the risks of future disadvantage. The chapters focused on two constituents of the transition, reviewing evidence on young people's educational and domestic trajectories. While the trajectories have been discussed separately, in reality they interlock. As this chapter has signalled, there is a dynamic interplay between, on the one hand, young people's educational and employment prospects and, on the other, their investment in routes into adulthood which do not depend on doing well at school and in the labour market.

Like young people's educational transitions to adulthood, domestic transitions are changing and polarizing. The chapter has drawn on both quantitative and qualitative studies to shed light on these changing transitions, looking particularly at pathways to early motherhood. Together, these sources of evidence suggest that young people, and particularly white young people, who enjoy the benefits of a well-off family and a good education, can use these resources strategically to protect their privileges. This requires that they defer entry into adult roles by remaining longer in the education system and outside cohabitation and parenthood. Young people without the resources acquired from their families and through the education system also use their adaptive capacities to develop life plans and strategies. But for them, plans and strategies are less about retaining their privileges and more about countering what Sennett and Cobb (1973) evocatively call 'the hidden injuries of class'. The example of young mothers suggests that formal modes of social participation (the student, the trainee, the paid worker) are less pivotal to these plans. Instead, it is informal modes of participation which can give meaning and direction to their lives. Young motherhood can bring not only a valued identity and a rewarding relationship, but can also maintain a female kin structure which is integral both to the mother's and her children's survival. However, while blunting the psychological and material impact of class disadvantage, this investment in early motherhood can serve to consolidate her disadvantaged position. It can also therefore mediate the intra-generational transmission of disadvantage, with the past and current circumstances of the mother shaping the conditions in which her children are born.

Chapter 10 turns the spotlight away from socio-economic inequalities to the health inequalities with which they are associated. It considers, in particular, how people's health is shaped by the circumstances in which they spend their formative years.

# 10 Health across unequal lives

## 10.1 Introduction

Chapter 7 introduced the concept of the social determinants of health and the conceptual frameworks that health researchers have developed to illuminate how these determinants shape people's health. The frameworks suggest that they originate in the social structure and work their way into people's environments and behaviours through the positions they occupy in this structure. Social position, and socio-economic position in particular, has therefore been identified as the pivotal determinant of health.

Identifying social position as pivotal suggests that socio-economic inequalities in health are the outcome of two sets of processes. First, there are mechanisms through which unequal positions are produced and maintained as people make their way through the social structure. Some mechanisms were examined in Chapters 8 and 9. The chapters looked particularly at the transition from childhood to adulthood, and pointed to the educational and domestic pathways along which advantage and disadvantage can pass from parents to children. Second, there are social and biological processes through which unequal positions become embodied in people's unequal health. Some of the processes are explored in Chapter 10. The word 'some' here is important: the research canvas is large and the chapter sketches in only a few aspects. It gives particular attention to evidence that people's health is influenced over and by the course of their lives. This 'life course perspective' is discussed in the section below. Building on the discussion, the chapter moves on to explore how circumstances in early life affect children's health. Introduced in Chapter 2, the concept of *developmental health*, signals that health is 'under development' in childhood, with the increase in children's physical, emotional and cognitive capabilities inseparable from what is popularly known as 'growing up'. The section takes foetal development, as measured by birth weight, and cognition, a term describing mental functions, such as thinking, learning and remembering. The penultimate section presents evidence on how people's socio-economic circumstances affect the biological processes of ageing. The concept of *functional ageing* draws attention to the capabilities whose rapid growth marked out the period of childhood, but this time in the context of decline. Functional ageing is therefore what is commonly called 'growing old'.

## 10.2 The socio-economic life course and health

Perspectives which emphasize that people's social biographies matter for their health go under the broad heading of 'life course perspectives'. These perspectives illuminate the ways in which people's past and current circumstances influence their health (Davey Smith *et al.*, 1997; Kuh *et al.*, 2003; Galobardes *et al.*, 2004). It is an approach which raises formidable methodological challenges. The temporal processes which link socio-economic conditions over generations and across people's lives are hard to unravel, as Chapters 8 and 9 have indicated. Hard to disentangle, too, are the mechanisms through which circumstances at different life stages – in childhood and adulthood, for example – influence people's health. Unravelling these connections is further constrained by the limited range of studies with information on circumstances in early and adult life. Most studies are of people born in the early- to mid-twentieth century in high-income countries – and in the UK, the Nordic countries and the USA in particular (Galobardes *et al.*, 2004). A number of studies only include men, with the difficulties of measuring women's socio-economic position further restricting analyses in which women are included (see Chapter 4, section 4.3). Like health inequalities research more broadly, life course analyses therefore draw heavily on evidence relating to middle-aged white men (Pollitt *et al.*, 2005).

In these analyses, the socio-economic life course is variously referred to as 'life course socioeconomic influences', 'the socioeconomic environment throughout life' and 'life course socioeconomic status' (Harper *et al.*, 2002: 396; Kuh *et al.*, 2004: 371; Pollitt *et al.*, 2005: 1). However it is characterized, the socio-economic life course is typically represented as the journey from the socio-economic environment of the natal family (usually indexed by father's occupation) to adulthood (own occupation). To investigate how this journey affects people's health, researchers have constructed longitudinal measures of people's socio-economic position using information collected at different time points. Figure 10.1 illustrates the patterns which emerge. It focuses on self-assessed health and is based on Britain's 1958 birth cohort study. The researchers combined data collected at four ages (birth, 16 years, 23 years and 33 years) into an overall socio-economic score (Power *et al.*, 1999). Those in the most advantaged circumstances (social classes I or II) at all four time points had a score of 4, a score which reached a maximum of 16 for those in the

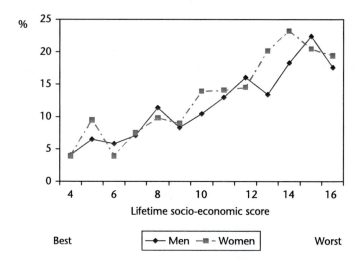

**Figure 10.1**   Poor health at age 33 by socio-economic circumstances (birth–33 years)

*Note:* Poor health is health assessed as poor or fair (rather than as good or excellent) health.

*Source:* Power, C. *et al.* (1999) The duration and timing of exposure: effects of environment on adult health, *American Journal of Public Health*, 89, 7, figure 1. Reprinted with permission from the American Public Health Association

poorest circumstances (social classes IV and V) at all four time points. As Figure 10.1 indicates, the proportion of the cohort who reported their health to be poor at age 33 rose in line with their exposure to poor circumstances. Among those whose lives had been spent in the best circumstances, under 5 per cent were in poor health; among the men and women who had been most exposed to disadvantage, rates of poor health reached nearly 20 per cent.

The relationship between lifetime circumstances and adult health captured in Figure 10.1 is not only evident for people in early adulthood. It is an association which continues into middle and old age. For example, a study which followed people through adulthood found a graded association between the duration of economic hardship and ill health. At the end of the 30 years of follow-up, rates of physical disease (diabetes, heart disease and cancer), clinical depression, physical impairment and poor cognitive functioning were at their lowest among those who never experienced economic hardship and climbed to their highest among those who never escaped it (Lynch *et al.*, 1997). As in other studies, the association between sustained hardship and poor health could not be explained by reverse causation: it was not the result of the onset of ill health causing subsequent economic hardship.

There is evidence that, like health outcomes, risk factors are also patterned by people's lifetime circumstances. Cigarette smoking, the major proximal determinant of poor health and premature death, provides an example. Most smokers take up the habit in their teenage years and the majority continue smoking into middle age (Schooling and Kuh, 2002; Jefferis *et al.*, 2004a). Childhood circumstances have been found to influence the odds of being an adult smoker, particularly for women (Schooling and Kuh, 2002; Jefferis *et al.*, 2004b; Power *et al.*, 2005). Current circumstances have a further and marked effect, with the result that rates of smoking are highest among adults who have experienced disadvantage across their lives (Jefferis *et al.*, 2004b; Power *et al.*, 2005).

Given the life course influences on health risks and health outcomes, it is not surprising to find that socio-economic circumstances across people's lives predict their chances of premature death. Figure 10.2 is based on a Scottish study of men aged 35 to 64. It uses information on father's occupation at birth, own occupation at entry into the labour market and occupation at the time of entry to the study to allocate men to a manual or non-manual social class at these three time points (Davey Smith *et al.*, 1997). As Figure 10.2 indicates, there is a graded association between cumulative social class and all-cause mortality. Thus, men in a manual social class at all three time points – the largest group – had the highest mortality rate over the 21 years of follow-up.

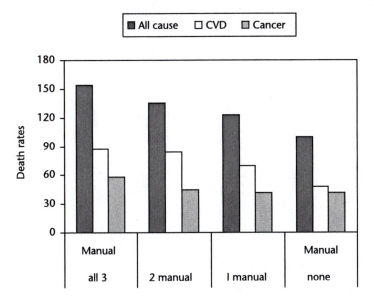

**Figure 10.2** Age-adjusted death rates (per 1000 person years) over 21 years of follow-up by cumulative social class, men age 35–64, Scotland: deaths from all causes, cardiovascular causes and cancer

*Note:* Social class based on non-manual/manual occupation at birth (father's job), first regular job and job at time of entry to study

*Source:* adapted from Davey Smith *et al.*, 1997, table 3

Mortality rates fell progressively for men who spent smaller proportions of their lives in the manual group. Death rates from cardiovascular disease and cancer revealed a similar pattern. Men born into, and remaining in, the manual group experienced the highest rates of death from these diseases; those in advantaged class positions in childhood and across adulthood had the lowest death rates from the 'big killers'. Conventional risk factors, like cigarette smoking and BMI, did not explain these different rates of death. The patterns revealed in Figures 10.1 and 10.2 suggest that 'lifetime' socio-economic position – measured from birth to adulthood – exerts a powerful influence on people's health. Analyses confirm that this is the case. Lifetime position emerges as a stronger predictor of adult disease and mortality risk than socio-economic position at any one point in time (Blane *et al.*, 1996; Davey Smith *et al.*, 1997).

While people's circumstances across their lives matter for health, there is evidence that childhood circumstances have particularly powerful effects (Galobardes *et al.*, 2004; Kuh *et al.*, 2004). Figure 10.3 describes the patterns for premature mortality. Based on the 1946 British birth cohort study, it plots the survival of children from manual and non-manual backgrounds from the age

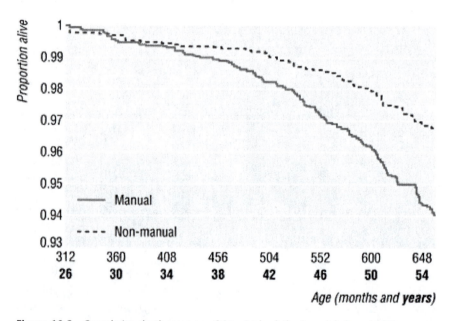

**Figure 10.3** Cumulative death rates age 26 to 54 by father's social class at birth among men and women in the 1946 birth cohort study

*Source:* Kuh, Hardy, Langenberg, Richards and Wadsworth, *British Medical Journal*, Nov. 9, 2002 (325: 7372) pp. 1076–80. Reproduced with permission of the BMJ Publishing group

of 26, when almost all children were still alive, to age 54. It captures the marked socio-economic differentials in survival, with death rates among women and men born into manual households double those of women and men growing up in non-manual households. Their increased risk of death was little reduced after account was taken of socio-economic circumstances in adulthood: in other words, the effect of poor circumstances in childhood was independent of whether adulthood brought continuing disadvantage or better circumstances (Kuh *et al.*, 2002). What is evident for all-cause mortality is repeated for a number of specific causes of death. For example, childhood disadvantage has been found to make a significant contribution to the risk of cardiovascular disease, over and above the effects of adult social class (Lawlor *et al.*, 2004). Childhood conditions are also independently linked to some cancers, like stomach cancer (Davey Smith *et al.*, 2001).

The patterns revealed in Figures 10.1 and 10.2 suggest that the trajectory which runs from parental occupation to own occupation has important effects on people's health. However, measuring the socio-economic life course only through people's relationship to the labour market obscures their position in the informal sphere of home and family, positions which are integral to women's socio-economic circumstances. For women, continuities in disadvantage from childhood to adulthood are importantly mediated by their reproductive and domestic careers (see Chapter 9). Extending the concept of the socio-economic life course to include these careers suggests that they play an important role in shaping the social distribution of health risks. Cigarette smoking provides an example. There are now a few studies which include both measures of the conventional socio-economic life course, like father's occupation and own occupation, and of women's domestic trajectories, like age at entry into motherhood and cohabitation status. These studies have found that early motherhood and lone motherhood increase the risk of adult smoking and reduce the odds of quitting, and do so over and above the effects of childhood disadvantage, educational disadvantage and poor current circumstances (Dorsett and Marsh, 1998; Graham and Der, 1999; Hobcraft and Kiernan, 2001; Jefferis *et al.*, 2004b; Rahkonen *et al.*, 2005).

A British survey provides illustrative evidence of the links between life course disadvantage and women's smoking status (Graham *et al.*, 2006a, 2006b). In Table 10.1, four markers of disadvantage are used: disadvantaged circumstances in childhood, early school leaving, early motherhood and severe adult disadvantage measured by reliance on means-tested welfare benefits. In the UK, these benefits provide an income appreciably below the EU poverty line (Ritakillio and Bradshaw, 2006). Table 10.1 plots the proportion of current smokers and quitters among women who experienced these cumulative forms of disadvantage (Graham *et al.*, 2006b). It begins with women who were disadvantaged in childhood. It then looks within this group at those who left school at the minimum school leaving age, narrowing the focus further to

**Table 10.1** Disadvantaged trajectories and smoking status of women aged 22 to 34, England, 1998–2002

|  | Current smoker | Ex-smoker (as % of ever smoker) |
|---|---|---|
| Childhood disadvantage[1] | 36 | 30 |
| + Left school ≤ 16 years | 44 | 28 |
| + Mother ≤ 21 years | 55 | 22 |
| + Adult disadvantage[2] | 63 | 17 |
| None of these | 18 | 45 |

*Notes*:
1  Father in routine/semi-routine occupation at birth or no contact with father.
2  On means-tested welfare benefits.

*Source*: adapted from Graham *et al.*, 2006b, table 1

women who also had their first baby by the age of 22. Finally, Table 10.1 records the rates of current smoking and quitting among young mothers who, additionally, were dependent on means-tested benefits. As it indicates, smoking prevalence rises and rates of cessation fall in line with increasing life course disadvantage. Among women from poor backgrounds who left school early, moved rapidly into parenthood and were on welfare benefits, 63 per cent were smokers. Among women with none of these disadvantages, prevalence rates stood at 18 per cent. While their smoking rates were much higher, only a small proportion (less than 5 per cent) of the women in the study had experienced these cumulative disadvantages: a much larger proportion (over a third) had avoided them all. As this suggests, information on the relative size of the disadvantaged group is important when thinking through the implications of evidence on their higher rates and higher risks of adverse outcomes (see Chapter 2, section 2.5).

Gendered trajectories of advantage and disadvantage matter for children, shaping the environments in which they develop, both *in utero* and after birth. The next section explores research which sheds light on how socio-economic trajectories are etched into their development.

## 10.3 Socio-economic inequalities in developmental health

The healthy development of children is a process beginning well before birth and which continues into the late teenage years. There is much that has yet to be learned about children's physical growth and cognitive development, as well as how they develop the secure sense of self needed to enjoy fulfilling social relationships and good psychological health. But three broad patterns are clear.

First, childhood marks a period of extraordinarily rapid development. It begins at the moment of conception and is at its most intense in the early months and years of life. The development process is genetically regulated and unfolds in a series of predictable and synchronized steps. But it is not genetically determined, driven only by genetic triggers and unmediated by the environment. Instead, child development – physical, cognitive, emotional and behavioural – is stimulated and shaped by the child's environment. It is therefore 'a complex and highly interactive process in which both biological regulation and experiential influences are substantial' (Shonkoff and Marshall, 2000: 35). As Box 10.1 notes, 'how genes are expressed is determined by a person's particular physical, psychological and social environment' (Halfon and Hochstein, 2002: 436).

Second, children may be more affected by their environment than adults, with experiences having a greater biological impact than they would in later life. The term 'sensitive period' is often used to signal the fact that childhood is a time of heightened sensitivity to environmental influences – and thus vulnerability to environmental adversity. In a sensitive period, 'an exposure has a stronger effect on development and subsequent disease risk than it would at other times' (Kuh *et al.*, 2003: 781).[1] The stronger effects happen because children's body systems are under development and therefore marked by considerable plasticity. Because of this plasticity, their bodies mould and adapt to the environments in which they are developing. The process is described as 'embodiment' and 'biological embedding' by epidemiologists (Kuh *et al.*, 2003). Experiences which are physically and emotionally nurturing become written into bodily structures and functions in ways which promote and protect their future health. Conversely, environmental adversity in the early years of life – chronic disadvantage, for example – has been found to induce long-term patterns of physical, cognitive and emotional development, which leave children vulnerable to developmental delay and poor health.

---

**Box 10.1**

'Some early "developmentalists" viewed human development as the unfolding of a genetically predetermined process of maturation and accordingly attributed less influence to environmental factors. More recent developmental theories place greater emphasis on the role of dynamic environment-gene transactions and on the mechanisms through which social contexts induce changes in psychological and biological functions ... That is, how genes are expressed is determined by a person's particular physical, psychological and social environment.' (Halfon and Hochstein, 2002: 436)

Third, as this suggests, inequalities in children's environments become 'written on the body'. There are of course genetic differences between children, and some of these differences are causes of developmental delay and future ill health (Mackenbach, 2005b). But genetic differences are not socio-economically patterned. They result from multiple combinations and interactions of genes, a complexity which 'makes it virtually impossible that the same genetic variants will be concentrated in any social class and transmitted more to children of that class than to the children of another class' (Holtzman, 2002: 535). What are socio-economically patterned, however, are environmental exposures which have biological consequences.

Separating environmental exposure from biological consequence is often not straightforward (Box 10.2). For example, social conditions in childhood may affect biological development, with these social and developmental factors combining to influence both social circumstances and health in later life. This interweaving of the social and the biological makes it difficult to attribute the effects of poor health in adulthood unambiguously to one or other set of mechanisms. With this complexity in mind, the section discusses the social patterning and health consequences of child development *in utero* and in the months and years after birth. It looks in particular at birth weight and cognition.

In the months from conception to birth, the environment in which the unborn child is living and growing is the mother's body and its effects on foetal development is indicated, although not entirely captured, by the baby's *birth weight*. Foetal development is influenced by the conditions of the mother's early life: by whether she was conceived and grew up in an environment which provided adequate nutrition to sustain her optimal growth and underwrite good health in adulthood (Perry and Lumey, 2004). The social class of grandparents therefore matters for the health of the child *in utero*. Foetal development is influenced, too, by the nutrient stores that the mother brings to the pregnancy and by her exposure to environmental toxins, like cigarette smoking, which increase the risk of preterm delivery and low birth weight (Kiernan and Pickett, 2006). This cluster of maternal factors is socially patterned (Kramer *et al.*, 2000). It is women who have faced a life time of disadvantage who are at greatest risk of poor health and nutritional

---

**Box 10.2**

'Research on life course and unequal health highlights the links between biological and social mechanisms. However, the difficulties of capturing the sequential complexities in crude statistical models means that caution is needed to avoid over-interpretation of findings'. (Power and Kuh, 2006: 47)

deficiencies; in high-income countries, they are also most likely to smoke and to smoke heavily (see Table 10.1 and Chapter 6, section 6.3).

Figure 10.4 plots the birth weights of UK babies born in 2000–1 by their mothers' social class as measured by the five-category NS-SEC (see Chapter 4, section 4.3). As it indicates, there are marked inequalities in this key dimension of developmental health. Mean birth weight is highest among babies born to mothers in the most advantaged circumstances (managerial and professional occupations), and falls in line with increasing socio-economic disadvantage (Dezateux *et al.*, 2004). The lowest mean birth weight is recorded by the babies of mothers in semi-routine and routine occupations. Birth weight, in turn, is an important determinant of infant survival and future health. Around 8 per cent of UK babies weigh less than 2500 grams at birth (defined as 'low birth weight') but this group accounts for over 60 per cent of deaths in the first year of life. In addition, there is strong evidence that birth weight influences cognitive development, with average performance in cognitive tests improving with increases in birth weight, and doing so independently of childhood circumstances (Jefferis *et al.*, 2002; Richards *et al.*, 2002).

The work of David Barker, a British epidemiologist, has been particularly important in stimulating interest in the developmental origins of adult health (Barker, 1998). He has suggested that poor maternal health and nutrient status

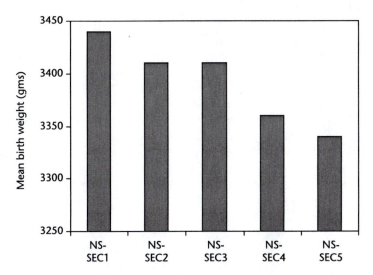

**Figure 10.4** Average (mean) birth weight by socio-economic circumstances at birth (NS-SEC of mother)

*Note:* NS-SEC based on main respondent: for the vast majority of babies, this was the natural mother.

*Source:* adapted from Dezateux *et al.*, 2004, table 7.34

result in foetal adaptations to under-nutrition. These adaptations help survival in the short term but 'may permanently change or "programme" the structure and function of the body' (Barker, 1997: 96). Barker has hypothesized that this process of foetal programming puts the child at heightened risk of being thin and small at birth – and of chronic disease in later life, like coronary heart disease and diabetes. Barker's hypothesis that disease-risk is prenatally programmed has not gone unchallenged, with researchers regarding it as focusing too narrowly on nutritional deficiencies and on the time window of pregnancy. But many agree with its underlying assumption that conditions in early life leave what Barker calls 'lasting memories' on children's body systems and therefore on their future health (1997: 96). Measuring the longer-term effects of poor foetal health requires longitudinal studies which have information on socio-economic circumstances in early and later life. The few analyses of birth weight which have included this information suggest that low birth weight is an independent risk factor for the development of cardiovascular disease (coronary heart disease and stroke) (Lawlor *et al.*, 2004). There is also evidence that the combination of poor foetal growth and subsequent weight gain is particularly important in increasing the risk of coronary death in adulthood: being overweight and obese increases the risk for everyone but especially for those who were born small (Rich-Edwards *et al.*, 2005).

*Cognitive development* provides an example of how the post-natal environment has biological consequences. Children come into the world with a rich network of brain cells already in place. But this neural network is activated and shaped by experiences after birth. At its most intense in the early months of life, this sculpting process continues apace through the pre-school years – and more slowly through later childhood and adolescence (Boyce and Keating, 2004). While there is still much to learn about how children's social environments influence the biology of brain development, there is evidence that they affect the skills which underpin learning – like verbal skills, problem-solving and memory. In turn, 'cognitively strong children will profit far more from any given curriculum and teaching than will their weaker counterparts' (Esping-Andersen, 2004: 229). It is a profit likely to be pay dividends in terms of higher qualifications and better job prospects. The effects of the early environment on cognitive development may therefore be an important factor in the transmission of inequalities in socio-economic position across generations (Machin and Vignoles, 2004).

A key source of insight into children's social environments comes from the thin seam of sociological studies of parenting. As earlier chapters have noted, these studies suggest that children's access to environments which nurture the development of cognitive skills is powerfully influenced by their family background. Parents moving through life on advantaged trajectories are well placed to furnish their children with a rich developmental environment: a materially secure home environment where they, or well-qualified substitute carers, organize activities which facilitate their children's cognitive development, as well as a school environment adapted to their individual educational needs. A lifetime of socio-economic disadvantage militates against this resource-intensive and child-centred approach to parenting. Parents in poorer circumstances are more likely to have been brought up in families facing financial hardship and to be experiencing continuing hardship in their adult lives, circumstances which can leave them depressed and unconfident about their parenting skills (Meadows and Dawson, 1999). Single and isolated risk factors appear to have little negative effect on child development: it is when children experience multiple risk factors that their cognitive development appears to suffer (Sameroff *et al.*, 1993). The message from research is that social disadvantage can put barriers in the way of children developing to their full potential, leaving them more vulnerable to developmental difficulties than their better-off contemporaries (Emerson *et al.*, 2006).

Figure 10.5 captures the socio-economic patterning of cognition among school aged children aged 7 to 16 years. It uses their scores in mathematics tests to measure cognition, mapping the scores for children from the most advantaged class backgrounds (parents in social classes I and II) and least

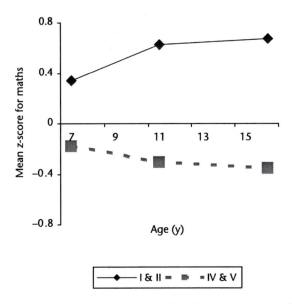

**Figure 10.5**    Mean z-scores for maths from ages 7 to 16 by social class at birth

*Note:* Excludes low birth weight children; social class IV and V includes children with no male head of household; and z-score of 0 is the average for that age; an increasing z-score with age indicates improvement in relative achievement.

*Source:* Jefferis, Power and Hertzman, *British Medical Journal*, Feb. 26, 2002 (325; 7359) p. 305–8. Reproduced with permission of the BMJ Publishing group

advantaged backgrounds (social classes IV and V) (Jefferis *et al.*, 2002). Because low birth weight increases the chances of neurological problems and cognitive impairment, children who weighed less than 2500 grams at birth are excluded. At each age, a score of 0 (marked by the horizontal line in Figure 10.5) is the average for the age group. A score which increases as the child gets older signals an improvement in their relative achievement; a declining score indicates that they are slipping further and further behind their peers. As Figure 10.5 suggests, the cognitive trajectories of children from richer and poorer families diverge as they move through the education system: it appears that children from professional families gain more from what schools are teaching and tests are assessing than their poorer contemporaries (see Chapter 8, section 8.5).

These data refer to British children born in 1958. What is the evidence for children today? Has the raft of changes introduced into the British educational system since this cohort was at school narrowed inequalities in cognitive development? The educational assessments which children in schools in England are required to undertake at ages 7, 11 and 14 years provide data which helps to answer this question. Modest inequalities in the mathematics scores of children from poorer and richer families are evident at age 7. By age 11 these inequalities have widened sharply, and increase further by the time of the final assessment at age 14 (DfES, 2006). As this suggests, contemporary patterns mirror those in Figure 10.5, with children's social backgrounds appearing to matter more rather than less for their cognitive development and educational success as they get older.

## 10.4 Socio-economic inequalities in functional ageing

Surveys of older people make clear that the majority are positive about the ageing process in general and about their health in particular. In England, over 70 per cent of those aged 60 and over feel younger than their years, and most – including people aged 80 and over – describe their health as good, very good or excellent (Demakakos *et al.*, 2006). But for most people the ageing process brings a decline in functional ability, with rates of physical impairment (like difficulty in walking) and cognitive impairment (like poor memory) increasing with age. As Guralnik *et al.* put it, 'midlife functional decrements are the beginning of a process of functional decline that results in high disability rates at old age' (2006: 700). Surveys point, too, to a progressive and age-related deterioration in self-assessed health across adulthood, with a steeper rate of decline for each passing year in older than younger age groups (Sacker *et al.*, 2005).

These trajectories of decline are socio-economically patterned. It is a patterning evident in both the timing and the speed of the ageing process. Health status starts to decline at younger ages among those in lower socio-economic groups (Sacker *et al.*, 2005). Impairment also progresses more rapidly in older people in poorer circumstances (Grundy and Glaser, 2000). In a study of men followed-up from the age of 45 to 65, the level of incapacity experienced by those in social class V by their mid-fifties was not reached by men in social class I until their mid-sixties (Gubéran and Usel, 1998). As other studies have found, functional ageing begins around ten years earlier in poorer groups, with men and women in disadvantaged circumstances ageing more quickly than their better-off contemporaries (Box 10.3).

Inequalities in the ageing process are reflected in rates of chronic disease like heart disease and respiratory illness which climb in line with declining social class among older men and women (McMunn *et al.*, 2003). It also means that the prevalence and severity of impairment is higher in lower socio-economic groups. This pattern is illustrated in Figure 10.6. It is based on the English Longitudinal Study of Ageing and focuses on physical impairment using an index discussed in Chapter 2, section 2.4. The index, the Short Physical Performance Battery, combines three dimensions of functioning: standing up from a sitting position, balance when standing and walking speed. Rates of impairment among those aged 60 and over are plotted by wealth, a measure which includes financial assets, pensions and property. As it suggests, the proportion living with physical impairments is at its lowest among the richest group and at its highest among the poorest groups: among women in the lowest wealth decile, 40 per cent are physically impaired (Melzer *et al.*, 2006).

People's lifetime experiences lie behind the patterns captured in Figure 10.6, with studies suggesting that socio-economic circumstances in early life have lasting effects on health in adulthood. Thus, childhood circumstances continue to be a significant predictor of physical and cognitive functioning through adulthood and into middle age (Richards and Wadsworth, 2004; Guralnik *et al.*, 2006). There is evidence, too, that socio-economic conditions in childhood are associated with risk factors for chronic disease, like higher

---

**Box 10.3**

'Ill health comes to us all eventually, but it comes, on average, at an earlier age to people lower down the social hierarchy. A similar pattern is evident for loss of function . . . There is a suggestion that the variation in the social inequality in health by age is a consequence of those in routine and manual occupational classes reaching a poor state of health a decade or two earlier in their lives than their peers in more advantaged positions. Around a third of men in the 50 to 59 age group report a limiting long-standing illness, while rates for men in professional and managerial groups remain much lower than this until they get beyond the age of 75'. (Marmot *et al.*, 2003: 5 and 209)

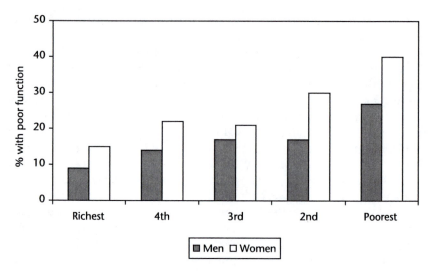

**Figure 10.6** Impairment on Short Physical Performance Battery score ≤ 8 by wealth quintile, adults aged 60 and over, England, 2004–5

*Source:* adapted from Melzer *et al.,* 2006,table 6A.10

BMI and higher diastolic blood pressure (Power *et al.,* 2007). The toll that early life disadvantage takes on adult health is captured in Figure 10.3, with higher death rates among adults from poorer backgrounds.

## 10.5 Conclusions

Earlier chapters have noted how a social gradient in health is evident at all stages of life. Figures and tables have illustrated that people's current health is related to their current circumstances in the early years, through childhood, and across early adulthood and older age. Life course perspectives extend the time frames for understanding these relationships. They suggest that cross-sectional associations between people's circumstances and their health are best understood as dynamic processes, with both circumstances and health shaped over time and across people's lives. As a result, social conditions in childhood influence both people's class position and their health status in adulthood and old age.

Mapping how social and biological processes are woven together as children grow up and adults grow old is a complex task. Social and health researchers have begun this cartographic project but still have some way to go. However, what is clear from the work undertaken so far is that the early years of life are a period of intensive development. In consequence, children, both before and after birth, are uniquely sensitive to environmental influences.

Family background plays an important role in shaping these environmental influences. Children born into socio-economic advantage are more likely to move along advantaged developmental trajectories. On average, they are heavier at birth, grow more quickly and end up taller than their less advantaged peers. Again on average, their cognitive development is more rapid and, at any given age, their cognitive skills are greater. They experience fewer behavioural difficulties and their psychological health is better. Conversely, children born into disadvantage can 'begin their lives with a poorer platform of health' (Najman *et al.*, 2004: 1147). Both their physical growth and their cognitive development can be compromised, with the latter identified as crucial for their confidence and progress at school. Inequalities in developmental health have major consequences for children's adult lives. They can feed into broader inequalities in children's social and health trajectories, which together increase the risk of both poverty and early onset of impairment and illness. By middle age, class inequalities appear to be already deeply etched into the ageing process. Both early life disadvantage and current disadvantage are linked to an earlier and more rapid decline in health. As sociologists have noted, 'the body is the most ubiquitous signifier of class' (Skeggs, 1997: 82; see Chapter 3, section 3.4).

In interpreting the evidence on the development and decline of health, it is important to remember that a much higher risk of an adverse outcome for children in disadvantaged groups – of low birth weight, for example – does not mean that it will inevitably occur. The outcome may well be rare even for children with the poorest start in life. What a higher risk suggests, however, is that poorer children are more vulnerable than children in more advantaged families to poorer outcomes. More broadly, it indicates that children's chances of fulfilling their developmental potential are unequal, with these chances determined by their family circumstances: by who their parents happen to be.

Inequalities in people's opportunities for optimal development in childhood and for functional health in adulthood are widely regarded as unjust and unfair. For many people, they represent what Rawls calls 'especially deep inequalities [which] cannot possibly be justified by an appeal to the notions of merit and desert' (1999: 7). These inequalities in development and ageing raise questions about the role of governments in moderating inequalities in people's circumstances. It is to the question of policy that the next chapter turns.

# 11 Unequal lives: policy matters

## 11.1 Introduction

Social and health research relies on surveys of individuals. As earlier chapters have noted, these surveys shed more light on the micro and proximal processes than on the macro and structural processes which underlie social and health inequalities. Nonetheless, they provide indirect evidence of the importance of these macro and structural factors. Data on individuals suggest that policies, and the societal institutions which they regulate, are an important part of the story of people's unequal lives.

This was the conclusion of the global and historical review of health inequalities undertaken in Part 2. It noted that the relationship between a country's wealth and health is mediated by policy; specifically it is mediated by what Tony Atkinson calls 'the redistributive ambitions of the government' (Atkinson, 1999: 286). Poor countries which harness their limited wealth to improve the social conditions of poor groups can achieve high life expectancies, while rich countries, like the USA, whose governments do less to equalize people's living standards have lower life expectancies than their wealth would predict. The importance of policy has been signalled, too, in Part 3. Chapter 7 noted the pivotal place of socio-economic position in the social processes which underlie health inequalities. It is a determinant whose constituent elements are policy sensitive: what governments do and do not do have major effects on people's educational opportunities, their employment and earnings, and their income and wealth. Chapters 8, 9 and 10 explored what inequalities in these core dimensions of socio-economic position mean for children, describing how children's unequal starting places contribute to inequalities in their future social and health trajectories. Here again, policy has a critical role to play.

Building on this evidence, the chapter focuses on the political and policy domains. It sets the scene by discussing contemporary public health policies, noting the priority given to reducing health inequalities and the emphasis placed on tackling their underlying determinants. Section 11.2 suggests that these tasks tend to be narrowly defined, with new initiatives targeting behavioural risk factors in poor groups. Less attention has been given to mainstream policies and how they work to maintain or to moderate the unequal distribution of wider determinants across the socio-economic hierarchy.

The central sections of the chapter turn to these broader policy effects. Section 11.3 looks at the welfare systems developed in high-income countries and their impact on inequalities in socio-economic position. Section 11.4 is concerned with the trend towards widening inequalities, and explores the extent to which its causes are beyond the influence of governments. In both sections, income inequalities are taken as the indicator of socio-economic position. This is because income inequalities serve as the most widely used metric through which the redistributive impact of government policies is measured. From a health perspective, income inequality provides a highly relevant metric. Income inequalities are the major determinant of people's unequal living standards and are, in turn, shaped by inequalities in education and occupation. Further, there is evidence that wide income inequalities take an additional toll on overall levels of health (Wilkinson and Pickett, 2006). Richard Wilkinson argues that this is because societies with marked income inequalities are characterized by less trust and less community spirit, dimensions which in turn lead to more violence, greater stress and poorer health (Wilkinson, 2005).

## 11.2 Policy approaches to tackling health inequalities

At both national and international level, the past three decades have seen major developments in public health policy. The traditional concern with improving overall levels of health has given way to a broader policy vision. This broader vision commits national governments and international agencies to tackling health inequalities. Thus, the international community has agreed that 'all governments must tackle poor health and inequalities as a matter of urgency' (WHO, 2005: 4). Reducing health inequalities has been identified as a target at European level. Europe has declared that 'the health gap between socio-economic groups within countries should be reduced . . . by substantially improving the level of health of disadvantaged groups' (WHO Europe, 1998: 1). At the national level, addressing health inequalities has been put at the centre of policy in an increasing number of countries both in Europe and beyond (see Chapter 7, section 7.2). 'Health inequalities' is often used as shorthand for the unequal distribution of health, although in some countries 'health disparities' is used instead (see Chapter 1, section 1.2). Thus, in the UK, the goal is to reduce health inequalities; in the USA, it is to reduce health disparities.

The goal of what the Swedish government calls 'good health on equal terms' is to be achieved by tackling the determinants of health. At international level, the 1998 World Health Assembly committed the member states of the WHO to 'addressing the basic determinants of health', a commitment reinforced at European level by an emphasis on 'multisectoral strategies to tackle the determinants of health' and 'the root causes of socio-economic inequities' (WHO Europe, 1998: 2, 9 and 14). At national level, England's public health policy is targeting both 'determinants of health' and 'determinants of health inequalities' (DoH, 2002: 22–3). Meanwhile, Northern Ireland's 'new approach to public health' is focused on 'the root causes of ill-health' and 'the root causes of health inequalities' (Secretary of State for Northern Ireland, 1999: 2; DHSSPS, 2000: 6). Basic determinants and root causes require attention because the factors which determine people's health are social not clinical (Box 11.1). As Sweden's public health strategy notes, they are 'factors in society or our living conditions that contribute to good or bad health' (Ågren, 2003: 5).

Chapter 7 discussed the models that health researchers have developed to explain these social factors to the policy community. In their different ways, these models make clear that health is the outcome of social processes beginning in the social structure and running through social positions to environmental and behavioural factors (see Figure 7.3). In line with these models, policy documents highlight 'smoking, alcohol abuse, nutrition, obesity, exercise', proximal factors that are linked to 'determinants such as income, education and employment' (Wanless, 2003: 24 and 33). As England's policy documents note, 'a wide range of government policies is needed to address the causes of health inequalities' (Box 11.1).

The UK is seen to be at the forefront of policy development. A review of

---

**Box 11.1**

'Poverty is the biggest risk factor for health, and income-related differences in health – which stretch in a gradient across all levels of the social hierarchy – are a serious injustice and reflect some of the most powerful influences on health . . . It is therefore imperative that public health policies address the root causes of socioeconomic inequities, and that fiscal, educational and social policies are designed to ensure a sustained reduction of health inequalities.' (WHO Europe, 1998: 14)

'Health inequalities are not just a health service issue. Many of the major determinants of health lie beyond the reach of the NHS [National Health Service], in people's living and working conditions and their health-related behaviours. The Programme For Action [England's public health strategy] reflects the recognition that a wide range of government policies is needed to address the causes of health inequalities.' (DoH, 2005: 14)

policies in Europe from 1990 to 2001 concluded that 'the UK, after a period of lagging behind continental Europe, now is ahead in development and implementation of policies to reduce socio-economic inequalities in health', noting that it is the only country which is moving towards 'comprehensive coordinated policy' (Mackenbach *et al.*, 2003: 1409). In an update of this review, European countries have been placed along a continuum, from those without a policy focus on health inequalities to those with integrated plans for addressing them. England and the devolved administrations of the UK dominate the latter group (Judge *et al.*, 2005).

In England, targets have been set for reducing health inequalities in life expectancy and infant mortality by 2010 and progress towards them is monitored (DoH, 2005, 2006). A raft of initiatives has been launched, with programmes for schools and local communities introduced alongside interventions for those at risk of long-term disadvantage (see Asthana and Halliday, 2006, ch. 2 for an overview). Many of the initiatives can be understood in life course terms. They seek to tackle the transmission of social and health disadvantage across generations and over people's lives: for example, by improving material conditions for poor children (Child Poverty strategy), their developmental health (Sure Start) and their transition to adulthood (Teenage Pregnancy strategy). Together, the package of interventions represents a significant advance on the policies of the 1980s and early 1990s.

However, the interventions have characteristics which are likely to weaken their impact on health inequalities. Their primary concern is with improving determinants in the poorest groups rather than with tackling the unequal distribution of determinants across the wider socio-economic hierarchy. The difficulty with such an approach is that positive changes in the target groups can be outpaced by faster rates of improvement in better-off groups. Britain's child poverty strategy provides an example. Between 1998 and 2005, the government achieved a marked decline in the proportion of children in poverty (in households below 60 per cent of median income) 'both through its decision to increase substantially the amount of cash transfers made to families with children and through welfare-to-work and other policies that have helped parents in previously workless families to find work and therefore increase their incomes' (Brewer *et al.*, 2006: 58). But the targeted approach gave little purchase on incomes higher up the income ladder. These continued to rise sharply, particularly at the upper end of the distribution, and the government missed its target of reducing the rate of child poverty by a quarter between 1998–9 and 2004–5 (Brewer *et al.*, 2006).

As this suggests, the effects of targeted interventions can be blunted by broader trends. This can be a particular problem for initiatives designed to reduce proximal risk factors like health behaviours and parenting practices. A common finding is that behavioural interventions are associated with widening rather than narrowing inequalities in the targeted risk factor. Box 11.2

---

**Box 11.2**

---

Evaluation of England's smoking cessation services: 'overall more disadvantaged groups tended to have lower cessation rates, ranging from 17.4% for group 1 (most advantaged) to just 8.7% for group 6 (most disadvantaged)'. (Ferguson *et al.*, 2005: 63)

Evaluation of the US's campaign to reduce deaths from Sudden Infant Death Syndrome (SIDS) by encouraging parents to put their babies on their backs to sleep: 'social class inequalities in SIDS did not narrow after the Back to Sleep campaign compared with the precampaign era. Although absolute risk of SIDS was reduced for all social class groups, a widening social class inequality was evident; women with more education have experienced a greater decline than women with less education'. (Pickett *et al.*, 2005: 1979)

Interim evaluation of England's Sure Start local programmes (SSLPs) designed to enhance the health and development of children under 4 years living in disadvantaged communities: 'SSLPs seem to benefit relatively less socially deprived parents (who have greater personal resources) but seem to have an adverse effect on the most disadvantaged children'. (Belsky *et al.*, 2006: 1476)

---

provides examples of this pattern. The problem may lie in the interventions themselves: it is possible that they are poorly designed, poorly delivered and underfunded. However, even an exemplary intervention will struggle to reduce inequalities in behavioural factors in the face of inequalities in factors higher up the causal chain. Analyses of persistent smoking among low-income households suggest that it is the persistence of disadvantage which holds the key to understanding why their cessation rates do not match the rates of success achieved in better-off groups (Dorsett and Marsh, 1998; Graham *et al.*, 2006b). Policies which reduce inequalities in life chances and living standards may therefore be a precondition for progress in reducing inequalities in proximal risk factors.

The next two sections focus on policies with the potential to moderate inequalities in these wider determinants. They look particularly at the extent to which welfare policies reduce inequalities in income between poorer and richer households.

## 11.3 Welfare systems and socio-economic inequalities

Until the twentieth century, high-income countries had limited systems for safeguarding the welfare of their populations. In the 1890s, public expenditure in the UK represented less than 10 per cent of gross domestic product, of which nearly half was for military and war-related expenditure (Le Grand, 1982). Governments played only a minimal role in regulating the workings of the economy and there was little publicly funded welfare provision, either in cash (like welfare benefits and state pensions) or in kind (like health care and education). But as the twentieth century progressed, state regulation of the labour market increased and the proportion of public expenditure devoted to welfare benefits and services rose. It was a trend that was particularly marked from the 1950s to the 1970s. By the end of the 1970s, public expenditure on welfare – devoted principally to income maintenance programmes, health care services, education and housing – represented 25 per cent of GDP in the UK. Elsewhere in Europe, welfare spending was higher still, reaching over 33 per cent of GDP in Denmark, Sweden and the Netherlands. Even in the USA, government spending on welfare services increased markedly, climbing to 20 per cent of GDP by 1980 (Therborn, 1989).

The strongly upward trend in welfare expenditure from 1950 to the late 1970s reflected a broad political consensus between right-leaning conservatives and left-leaning socialists. While there were dissenting voices in many countries, the centre ground agreed that interventionist economic and social policies were unavoidable. This was because unregulated markets were not delivering the employment conditions and the welfare services that rich economies needed in order to grow and that their populations needed in order to prosper. More active government control of the economy was therefore one part of the consensus; the other was better collective mechanisms to enable people to 'fare well' across their lives. These collective mechanisms constitute what is often referred to as a welfare state. Definitions vary, but its key feature is that it provides people with essential resources independently of their economic circumstances (see Box 11.3). Core elements include systems to maintain people's incomes when the market fails to provide for them – during unemployment and old age, for example – and services like education and health care 'without which nobody can be guaranteed a decent life in a modern society' (Miller, 2003: 105). These systems of cash benefits and welfare services are funded by taxation in various forms: direct taxes on earnings and investments, indirect taxes on goods and services, and payroll taxes paid by workers and employers.

---

**Box 11.3**

'The welfare state [comprises] the set of institutions and policies that distribute both money and essential goods and services to citizens on a non-market basis.'
(Miller, 2003: 95)

Welfare states, along with the tax systems which fund them, have major effects on the distribution of resources across people's lives. Specifically, they protect living standards and meet welfare needs at periods in the life course when the individual is most vulnerable, by transferring resources from periods where he or she is earning and in good health. The transfer process works by collecting funds from working-age adults in the form of taxes, and paying them out in the form of cash benefits and welfare services to the non-working generations. Thus, taxes and benefits smooth out income between childhood (when the individual is too young to work and pay tax), adulthood (when they are likely to be doing both), and older age (when again they are likely to be outside the labour market). Welfare services, too, have a strong life course orientation, with expenditure and utilization concentrated in younger and older age groups. The largest budgets are for education and health care, and in all welfare systems children are the major users of education and older people are the major consumers of health care (Ginsberg, 1993; Sefton, 2002). Taken together, direct taxes, cash benefits and welfare services are highly redistributive, 'succeeding in the aim of adding incomes at times of "want" through transfers from the times of "plenty"' (Falkingham and Hills, 1995a: 101). In the UK, reducing inequalities in income at different points in the individual's life is the major redistributive effect of the welfare state: the scale of intra-personal redistribution is much greater than that between individuals (Falkingham and Hills, 1995b).

While redistribution across age groups and life stages has been an accepted objective of welfare systems, support for broader social distribution has been more muted. For those on the conservative side of the welfare consensus, the concern has been with maintaining, rather than eroding, existing status differentials. On this side of the consensus, redistribution is usually seen in minimal terms. The preference is for economic policies which do little to alter the earnings gap between lower and higher paid workers, and a welfare state which provides a basic safety net for the poorest groups. In the USA – where the ideology of minimal intervention is so deeply entrenched that politicians are reluctant to describe the welfare system as a welfare state – means-tested benefits are designed to save those who meet the strict eligibility criteria from destitution. At the left-leaning end of the consensus, redistribution tends to be seen in broader terms. In the Nordic countries, for example, there is an emphasis on strong labour market policies to contain earnings inequalities and a welfare state which provides 'equality of the highest standards' across socio-economic groups and between men and women (Esping-Andersen, 1990: 27). Here the tax and welfare systems are seen as a mechanism for promoting a more egalitarian society: pooling resources by means of taxation and using 'the funds thus obtained to make accessible to all, irrespective of their income, occupation or social position, the conditions of civilization which, in the absence of such measures, can be only enjoyed by the few'

(Tawney, 1931: 122). It is an aim in accord with Rawls's vision of a just society in which people's moral equality is expressed by everyone having access to a core set of primary social goods (see Chapter 1, section 1.3).

The UK combines features of both approaches. The 1940s established a welfare state in which secondary education and health care were to be provided on a universal basis. School education was made free for all children and the National Health Service removed almost all charges for medical care through services designed to 'universalize the best' (see Chapter 5, section 5.4). However, the social security system was not refashioned on these universal principles. It has continued to provide a safety net of means-tested benefits set below the poverty line and therefore 'reserved for the poor' (Deacon and Bradshaw, 1983).

While the UK welfare system, like those in most high-income countries, was not designed to reduce social inequalities, it is often judged in these terms (Powell, 1995). Assessing the equity effects of welfare states is not an easy task. It requires reliable measures of both policy inputs and welfare outputs, measures which are hard to find for constituents of socio-economic position like education and employment. Income inequalities have therefore been a major focus. Analyses compare the magnitude of inequality in market income (before direct taxes are deducted and welfare benefits received) and disposable income (after these income transfers), with the difference between the two serving as an indicator of the redistributive effects of welfare systems. Because of differences in methodologies, the findings of different studies are often not directly comparable (Atkinson *et al.*, 1995).

There are other limitations with this approach. Focused on income, it misses the contribution of inequalities in private wealth, like home ownership, to inequalities in living standards. It misses, too, the redistributive impact of policies which work through equalizing market incomes, for example, through minimum wages. It also fails to take account of redistribution through the provision of services in kind, like education and health care; however as discussed below, the approach can be extended to investigate these distributive effects. In addition, caution needs to be exercised when attributing differences in the distribution of market and disposable income to tax and benefit policies. Factors other than the tax and benefit systems will also play a part (Ritakallio, 2002). However despite these limitations, some broad conclusions can be drawn.

There is evidence that welfare states reduce gender inequalities in income. In the UK, for example, inequalities in disposable income and living standards between men and women – and between lone motherhood households and two-parent households in particular – would be much more pronounced without the moderating effects of the welfare system. The reason is that men's lifetime earnings are, on average, twice those of women's, a gap which is significantly reduced when account is taken of tax and benefits. In consequence, 'overwhelmingly women are net gainers from the system and men are net losers' (Evandrou and Falkingham, 1995: 149). There is a larger pool of research on the impact of welfare policies on income inequalities between richer and poorer households. These analyses look at the effects of the three major instruments: taxes, cash benefits and welfare services.

### Taxes and cash transfers

Taxes on earnings are progressive: they take a larger share of the income of richer than poorer households. They therefore make inequalities in disposable income smaller than those in market incomes. But disposable income does not take account of indirect taxes. These taxes – on cigarettes and clothes, for example – are regressive, absorbing a larger proportion of the income of the poor. In the UK, progressive and regressive taxes cancel each other out, with the result that the overall tax system has virtually no effect on the magnitude of income inequalities (Jones, 2005). A similar pattern is evident in other high-income countries (Glyn, 2006). In contrast, cash transfers are pro-poor. Because welfare benefits are the major source of income for the poorest groups but represent only a very small proportion of the income of the rich, they reduce inequalities in market incomes (Harris, 2000; Palme *et al.*, 2003). In the UK, these cash benefits play the largest part in equalizing incomes and living standards (Harris, 2000; Jones, 2005).

Figure 11.1 provides evidence of the combined redistributive effects of direct taxes and cash transfers on households in the USA, the UK and Sweden (Ritakallio, 2002). It compares the proportion of households living in poverty (less than 50 per cent of median income) based on their market income and their disposable income. It is interesting to note that the market economies of all three countries leave their populations exposed to high levels of poverty. Without a tax and benefit system, nearly 30 per cent of households in the USA would be living in poverty; in the UK and Sweden, the proportion is higher still. Taxes and benefits reduce market-generated levels of poverty in all three countries. However, the effectiveness of these redistributive instruments varies. The Nordic system, with its more progressive tax system and its structure of universal benefits, is more efficient than the UK and US systems which rely on means-tested benefits targeted at the poorest households. In Sweden, the tax and benefit system achieves a 90 per cent reduction in the rate of poverty generated by the market. In the UK it is 66 per cent; in the USA it is 38 per cent (Ritakallio, 2002). While taxes and benefits reduce inequalities in income, they nonetheless remain pronounced. In the UK, the richest 20 per cent of households still have seven times as much to spend per year (around £42,000 in 2004) as the poorest 20 per cent of households (£6000) (Jones, 2005).

Studies of the redistributive impact of direct taxes and welfare benefits have paid particular attention to how they combine to moderate income inequalities in childhood. As Chapters 8, 9 and 10 have highlighted, child-

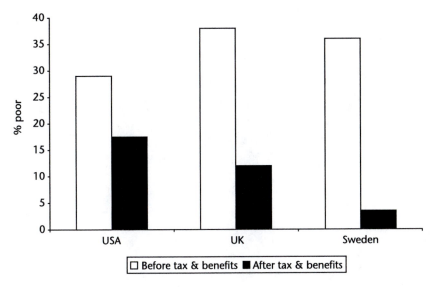

**Figure 11.1** Poverty rates (below 50 per cent of mean household income) before and after income transfers (direct tax and welfare benefits), 1995

*Source:* adapted from Ritakallio, 2002, figures 1 and 3

hood is a period of life when social conditions have powerful effects on social and health trajectories. It is also one of heightened vulnerability to poverty (UNICEF, 2005; Ritakallio and Bradshaw, 2006). National systems of tax and benefits vary in the extent to which they protect children's living standards. In some countries, these systems combine to lift a large proportion of children above the poverty line. In others, the systems appear to be less effective. Figure 11.2 illustrates these national differences by comparing child poverty rates before and after direct taxes have been deducted and cash benefits have been paid. These transfers reduce child poverty rates by over 70 per cent in Nordic countries like Sweden; in the UK, the reduction is 46 per cent and in the USA it is 19 per cent (Whiteford and Adema, 2006).

### Welfare services

Welfare services, like state education, health care, social housing and social care services, are a major component of government expenditure. In the UK, they consume about a third of public spending, with education and health care taking the lion's share (Sefton, 2002). Because they represent a substantial addition to people's cash incomes, these services are called 'the social wage' (Box 11.4). The value of the social wage for a household rises as its market incomes fall (Jones, 2005). This is because the major users of education and

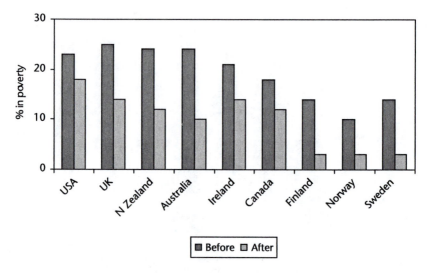

**Figure 11.2** Child poverty rates (below 50 per cent of median household income) before and after income transfers (direct tax and welfare benefits), 2000

*Source:* adapted from Whiteford and Adema, 2006, table 9

---

**Box 11.4**

'The social wage is a measure of how much better off individuals are with the provision of publicly-funded welfare services than they would be without these "in kind" services (that is, if they had to pay the full cost of these services).' (Sefton, 2002: 1)

---

health care – children and older people – are disproportionately found in poorer households. To illustrate the pro-poor bias of welfare services, estimates for Britain suggest that the average cost of providing health care, education and social housing was £1680 per person in 2000–1, ranging from £2100 for the poorest fifth of the population to £1010 for the richest fifth (Sefton, 2002).

Welfare services represent a higher proportion of the disposable income of poorer groups, underpinning their living standards to a much greater extent than for households further up the income distribution (Harris, 2000). This is illustrated in Figure 11.3. It represents the value of benefits in kind as a proportion of household income after direct taxes, cash benefits and indirect taxes have been taken into account (called 'post-tax income'). In non-retired households, these services have a cash value equivalent to nearly 90 per cent of the post-tax incomes of the bottom income quintile. For the richest quintile, they are equivalent to under 10 per cent of their income. As Figure 11.3 makes clear,

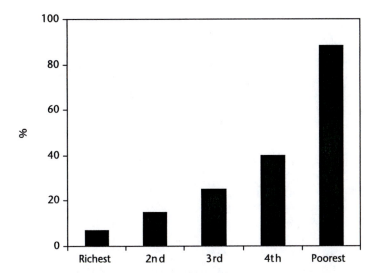

**Figure 11.3** Value of benefits in kind for non-retired households as a percentage of post-tax income by income quintile groups, UK, 1998–9

*Note:* Post-tax income takes account of cash benefits, direct taxes and indirect taxes; benefits include education, NHS, housing subsidy, travel subsidies, school meals and welfare milk.

*Source:* adapted from Jones, 2005, table 10

the social wage is pro-poor, providing a mechanism through which to level up access to essential goods and services.

The social wage can play a particularly important role in childhood, when the risks of disadvantage are higher and its long-term effects are greater than at other life stages. It can therefore serve to equalize access to the resources on which socio-economic advantage and good health are built. An example is investment in pre-school provision (Box 11.5). Greater equality of access to high-quality pre-school care has been identified as one reason why parental social class has weaker effects on children's cognitive development and on their educational attainment in Nordic countries than in other high-income

---

**Box 11.5**

'Day care in the United States is almost exclusively privately provided, and quality care is simply priced out of the market for low-income families. Scandinavian day care is basically of uniform, high pedagogical standards, meaning that children from disadvantaged families will benefit disproportionately. Day care in the United States is of extremely uneven quality, and children from disadvantaged families are concentrated at the low end.' (Esping-Andersen, 2004: 308)

countries, like the UK and the USA (Esping-Andersen, 2004). But equality of access may not be enough to achieve equality in what Sen calls substantive freedoms. Children from poorer backgrounds may require greater educational opportunities to gain the advantages which middle-class children derive from their years at school. However, evidence discussed in Chapters 3 and 8 suggests that they are struggling to secure an educational experience of the quality enjoyed by their better-off peers.

## 11.4 Widening income inequalities

The period from 1950 to the late 1970s was the heyday of what Tony Atkinson calls 'the redistributive state' (1999: 69). Across these decades, high employment combined with rising public expenditure to narrow income inequalities in the UK. In other high-income countries, including the USA, richer households saw their share of national income fall (Mishel *et al.*, 2006). Analyses suggest that income inequalities reached particularly low levels in Finland, Norway and Sweden (Atkinson *et al.*, 1995).

From the late 1970s, a different picture started to emerge. It was one first evident in the UK, and is captured in Figure 11.4. It plots the weekly disposable incomes of the poorest tenth and the richest tenth of households, pointing to marked but stable inequalities from the early 1960s to the late 1970s. From this point, real incomes at the upper end of the distribution set off on a sharply

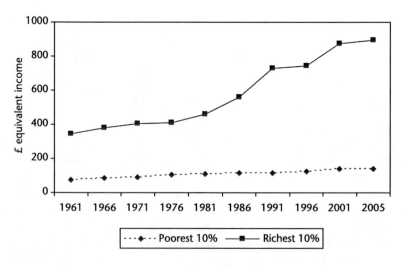

**Figure 11.4** Weekly household incomes of poorest and richest 10 per cent, before housing costs, Britain, 1961–2005

*Source:* adapted from IFS website

upward trajectory. The incomes of the poor, meanwhile, stagnated. Since the 1990s, inequalities in disposable income have continued to widen, but at a slower rate. Figure 11.4 provides the economic backdrop against which social and health inequalities have been reproduced in Britain over the past half-century. It is the context, too, in which the current drive to reduce health inequalities is set. It is perhaps not surprising that, to date, interventions which target proximal determinants are struggling to make a dent on inequalities in either the targeted risk factors or in health.

Widening income inequalities in Britain have had important life course consequences, with rates of poverty rising more steeply for children than for the population as a whole. In the late 1970s, overall poverty rates and child poverty rates were similar, standing at 13 per cent and 14 per cent respectively (based on a poverty line of 60 per cent of median income, after housing costs). By the early 1990s, one in four (24 per cent) of the population, and one in three (33 per cent) of children were in poverty. The child poverty rate has since declined from this peak. In 2005, 3.4 million children were living in households below the poverty line: 19 per cent of all children.

From the early 1980s, income inequalities started to rise in the USA, a country in which the gap between rich and poor was already markedly higher than in other high-income countries (Atkinson *et al.*, 1995). Subsequently, other countries have seen income inequalities widen, including New Zealand. But others have bucked the trend, with either no increases in income inequalities over the 1980s and 1990s or only recent and modest rises (Atkinson, 2002b; Lahelma *et al.*, 2002; Palme *et al.*, 2003). In Finland and Sweden, for example, the 1990s saw major economic shocks, with deep recessions and rising unemployment fuelling a significant increase in market income inequalities (Fritzell, 2001). However, inequalities in disposable income changed little and rates of poverty rates remained low. For example, the poverty rate (below 60 per cent of median household income) in Sweden was 7 per cent in 1990 and 8 per cent in 1999, with little difference in poverty rates between high-ranking salaried workers and manual workers (Palme *et al.*, 2003).

There are two rival interpretations of the income distribution in high-income countries. The first argues that a widening gap in the incomes of rich and poor is inevitable, a trend which will engulf all societies. This will happen because it is driven by external factors so powerful that they are overwhelming the redistributive capacities of welfare systems. In this perspective, the policy instruments available to nation states, like taxes, benefits and welfare services, are insufficient to moderate the polarizing effects of market forces (Atkinson, 2002b). Key among these market forces is a fall in the demand for manual and unskilled labour in countries which are making the transition from industrial to post-industrial societies (see Chapter 8, section 8.2). Globalization is seen to lie behind the fall in demand for low-skilled workers, with an increasingly competitive global market place determining – and thus limiting – what national governments can do. Their autonomy and influence is being squeezed to the point where their only function is to adapt their populations to the harsh realities of the global economy (Mullard, 2004).

The alternative interpretation is that widening inequalities in high-income countries are not inevitable. The diverging patterns of inequality between countries are cited as evidence for this view (Atkinson *et al.*, 1995; Smeeding, 2002). These comparative studies conclude that 'it is not the case that all countries are following a common pattern, despite the fact that the countries were exposed to the same forces of international competition and of technological change' (Atkinson, 1995: 63). What is seen as critical are not global forces but national policies, with the countries where income inequalities rose most steeply through the 1980s and 1990s – the UK, USA and New Zealand – led by governments that had moved decisively to the right. As noted in Chapter 8, section 8.2, the emphasis was on deregulating the labour market and reducing public expenditure because, as a leading government minister put it, 'cuts in state spending are essential to make way for the revival of the wealth-creating sector' (Joseph, 1977). In the UK, for example, policies during the 1980s weakened the power both of trade unions and of the mechanism to control minimum pay rates at the bottom of the earnings distribution and pay levels at the top. Policies also reduced the progressiveness of taxation and the scope and level of welfare benefits. In the UK, as in other countries which embraced right-wing policies, these have been identified as a major cause of the increases in income inequalities and child poverty which they have experienced (Atkinson, 2002; Dalziel, 2002; Goodman and Shepherd, 2002; Mishel *et al.*, 2006). As this suggests, government action and inaction play a major role in shaping the distribution of income (Box 11.6).

This alternative interpretation also draws attention to policy choices at the global level. Since the 1970s, the powerful players on the world stage – the USA, multinational corporations and international financial agencies – have favoured a particular form of global economic integration. This involves less government intervention in national labour markets and in welfare provision as well as fewer restrictions on foreign investment and trade (UNDP, 2005; Birdsall, 2006; Glyn, 2006). It is increasingly recognized that the costs and

---

**Box 11.6**

'Domestic policies – labour market institutions, welfare policies etc – can act as a powerful countervailing force to market driven inequality. Even in a globalised world, the distribution of income in a country remains very much a consequence of the domestic political, institutional and economic choices made by those individual countries – both rich and middle income ones.' (Smeeding, 2002: 28)

benefits of the approach 'have been unevenly distributed across and within countries, perpetuating a pattern of globalization that builds prosperity for some amid mass poverty and deepening inequality for others' (UNDP, 2005: 113). The dominance of this form of globalization is seen to have an additional and ideological effect, casting the deregulation of markets, cut backs in welfare provision and spiralling income inequalities as outcomes over which governments have no control. Against this view, it is argued that global economies, like national ones, are 'social constructs, fashioned, shaped and defined in the policy process' (Box 11.7).

---

**Box 11.7**

'Globalisation is at present being shaped and defined within the specific discourse of market liberalism. Implicitly, it is a discourse that encourages views about the limits of government and the retreat from the public space . . . Governments are not prisoners of globalisation. The major increases in capital flows in financial markets, decisions on world trade and deregulation of labour markets represent deliberate policy decisions. Markets are social constructs, fashioned, shaped and defined in the policy process.' (Mullard, 2004: xii and xiii)

---

As social constructs, economies can change. International agencies like the United Nations are increasingly arguing for policies which are explicitly pro-poor. In line with Sen's capabilities approach, they advocate national and global policies which equalize 'the opportunities that shape the distribution of income, education, health and wider life chances' (UNDP, 2005: 51).

## 11.5 Conclusions

Over the past ten years, public health policy at both national and international level has turned its attention to health inequalities. Policy goals have been reconfigured to give greater attention to tackling the social factors which underlie the unequal distribution of health. The UK has been at the forefront of this reorientation of public health policy. Here, as elsewhere, the new policies have taken a particular form. Attention has focused on improving the health of those in the poorest circumstances through interventions which target behavioural influences on their health. To date, there is little evidence that either inequalities in these behavioural factors or inequalities in health are narrowing. The lack of progress may reflect weaknesses in the interventions themselves. However, the problem may lie, alternatively or additionally, in the contexts in which the interventions are being introduced. Persisting and widening inequalities in people's socio-economic circumstances are likely to militate against the success of the downstream interventions through which the public health goal of greater health equality is being pursued.

The chapter has focused on policies which can exert an influence on the distribution of wider determinants. It has looked in particular at policies which influence the distribution of income. It noted their important life course effects, with the tax and welfare benefits systems smoothing out the distribution of income between childhood, adulthood and older age. The provision of services in kind (the social wage) also moves resources across the life course. However, taxes, cash benefits and welfare services do more than redistribute resources across people's lives. They also redistribute resources between rich and poor. The chapter presented evidence that taxes and benefits moderate market income inequality, leaving poorer households richer and richer households poorer than they would otherwise be. The extent to which they do so varies markedly between countries. In broad terms, political visions and moral values appear to matter. Countries with an explicit and enduring commitment to greater social equality have economic policies and welfare systems that are more effective at moderating the inequalities that markets produce. In countries without this commitment, policies and systems do much less to redistribute market wealth between richer and poorer households. These national differences appear to have survived the emergence of global labour markets and the increasing economic interdependence of nation states. Even in a globalizing world, national welfare systems remain distinctive in their size and structure – and thus different in their impacts on social inequalities.

# Concluding comment

'Health inequalities' is a term with a range of meanings. It is most commonly used to refer to differences in the health of people occupying unequal positions in the societies of which they are part. In particular, it is the term which describes the unequal health of unequal socio-economic groups. It is these socio-economic inequalities in health which have been the focus of the book.

Earlier chapters have documented how health inequalities exist when death rates are high and infectious disease takes a heavy toll on people's health. They are maintained as countries become wealthier and healthier, and chronic diseases emerge as the major cause of death. The persistence of health inequalities over time and despite changes in economic and health conditions suggests that disease-specific factors – like poor sanitation in poorer countries and cigarette smoking in richer ones – are unlikely to hold the key to understanding health inequalities. The explanatory models which health researchers have produced point, instead, to inequalities in wider determinants as underlying the enduring association between socio-economic position and health. What this suggests is that health inequalities have persisted because both the structures of society and the circumstances in which people live have remained unequal.

Looking particularly at high-income countries and taking the UK as a case study, *Unequal Lives* has investigated how the process works. The complexity of the process means that the book offers some insights: it is far from a complete analysis. Earlier chapters have explored social research which sheds light on how socio-economic inequalities endure across people's lives and epidemiological research which has investigated how these enduring inequalities become embodied in their health.

Research within the disciplines of sociology and social policy provide an important perspective on how socio-economic inequalities endure. It suggests that inequalities are both imposed by social structures and are fashioned by individuals.

With respect to structural factors, the book has discussed how labour markets and education systems provide resources that are essential for people to survive and prosper. But they do so in ways which stratify people: they assess people and allocate them to different and unequal locations in their structures. Welfare systems moderate socio-economic inequalities, for example, by opening up access to education for poorer groups and by reducing inequalities in market incomes. But the redistributive effects still leave people unequally placed in the socio-economic hierarchy. In the UK, for example, young people from poorer backgrounds gain less from the education system – and have gained less from its recent expansion – and the combined effects of the tax and benefit systems leave marked inequalities in disposable incomes.

With respect to the individual processes which generate inequalities, the chapters noted that social structures are not simply 'out there', lying in wait to catch people and force them into their allotted place in the pecking order. Sociological studies suggest that unequal positions are also being actively produced, routinely and day by day, as people go about their lives. Chapters have described how parents in advantaged positions deploy their economic and social privileges to help their children do well at school and secure entry to the higher echelons of the labour market. Domestic trajectories are integral to this process of social reproduction, particularly for women. Deferring motherhood and settling down with a partner with high earning potential helps women from advantaged backgrounds to consolidate their – and their children's – position on the higher rungs of the class ladder. For young people without the economic and cultural capital secured through an advantaged social background, it can be harder to do well at school and in the labour market. Many succeed; the odds, however, are lower than for young people from privileged backgrounds. Early motherhood and lone motherhood can make it more difficult to avoid long-term hardship, further reducing the chances of high lifetime living standards for parents and their children.

Drawing on evidence from social epidemiology, the book has explored how social inequalities become embodied in people's health. It has noted how advantaged circumstances, from childhood and across adulthood, are associated with better health. Conversely, poorer lifetime circumstances are associated with an earlier onset of ageing and a higher risk of chronic disease and premature death. Studies have drawn particular attention to the influence of conditions in early life. Epidemiologists have uncovered evidence that genetic processes which govern children's development are triggered by their environments; as a result, inequalities in children's circumstances can become embodied in their body structures and functions. Cognitive development provides an example of how inequalities in children's lives may become 'written on the body', with those growing up with professional and well-off parents being additionally advantaged by the extra economic and cultural capital that is typically invested in helping them do well at school. Conditions in childhood also influence people's body shape and health-related behaviours: social class is displayed through height and weight as well as through habits like cigarette smoking. As this suggests, sociological and epidemiological perspectives are converging in their focus on embodiment as a key process in the persistence of both social and health inequalities across people's lives.

When trying to make sense of social and health inequalities, researchers often compare the experiences of those in the poorest circumstances with those in the most advantaged positions. In many ways it is a helpful way of presenting the evidence. The comparisons bring out the magnitude of inequalities in people's incomes and living standards, even in rich countries where there is more than enough for all. Taking the best-off as the reference group captures the health disadvantages of being poor, pointing to higher risks of poor health from before birth and across the life course. But there are drawbacks to relying on comparisons between poor and rich to make sense of inequalities. It can be difficult for those who are not statisticians to appreciate that a higher risk of an adverse outcome does not necessarily mean that it is going to – or is even likely to – happen. Experiences found to have a negative impact on future socio-economic position and future health may not occur that often, even in the most disadvantaged group. Further, taking the best-off group as the reference category can imply that they are the normative group. In other words, they are not simply more privileged; their lifestyles are better. Such a perspective casts poorer groups as the problem: it implies that if they only modified their lifestyles and parenting practices to be more like richer groups, all would be well. It is a perspective which locates cause and solution at the 'downstream' end of the causal pathway. Such an approach leaves inequalities in upstream determinants intact and undisturbed. However, the evidence suggests that it is the persistence of these inequalities – inequalities in the structural institutions of society, like the labour market and in people's positions within them – which underlies the persistence of health inequalities.

These unequal structures and positions, and the health inequalities which flow from them, are widely regarded as unjust. As the United Nations observes, persisting inequalities in life chances and health chances, and inequalities stemming from inherited advantage in particular, violate basic precepts of social justice (UNDP, 2005: 12). It violates the principle that people are morally equal. This is the principle that everyone – and therefore everyone's life and everyone's health – matters equally. A society which honoured the principle would be appalled at the scale of social and health inequalities evident in rich societies, like the UK and across the world. It would seek to ensure that, at a minimum, everyone had an equal start in life and an equal chance of living a long and healthy life. Its aim would be for each of us, regardless of our place of birth and who our parents might be, to have equal basic freedoms.

Philosophy has shed an important light on the equal freedoms on which a just society would be built. Some philosophers suggest that these are best seen as equal inputs into people's lives, like equal political rights and an equal allocation of basic resources. Amartya Sen has made the case for a concept of freedom which puts less emphasis on inputs and gives more attention to outcomes: to the lives that people are able to lead and the standards of health they are able to achieve. It is a perspective which suggests that societies which seek to be just and fair will promote equality in what people can do and achieve. Central to this perspective is the recognition that children will require different kinds and quantities of inputs to achieve equality in their substantive freedoms as they grow up: for example, to fulfil their developmental potential and to enjoy good health in later life. Children are likely, too, to require different blends of resources and opportunities as they move through adulthood and grow older. Children who start life with less, by way of economic and social resources, should expect to receive more and different inputs than other children to enable all, whatever their circumstances, to build lives which they value equally.

It can, of course, be argued that imagining such a society is a pipedream: a vision of equality which could never be turned into reality. It is an argument which is often made. It suggests that moral visions can carry no political weight if they are difficult – or impossible – to achieve. It is an argument which rests on the view that, if something cannot be done, it cannot be claimed to be morally right to try to do it. The counter-position is that the difficulty of achieving an ethical outcome does not invalidate its moral force. Further, as the long struggles and campaigns against oppression have demonstrated, making the moral case for greater equality is integral to the process of securing social and political change. Making the moral case can awaken and articulate a social conscience. It can help to strengthen and mobilize public concern, to encourage political debate, to shame governments into action.

The recent history of national and global politics underlines how important a social conscience and moral vision is. Over the last 30 years, the political consensus which recognized that governments need to be actively engaged in the management of market economies and in the provision of welfare services has fragmented. The right-leaning side of the consensus has gained ascendancy in an increasing number of countries. This favours a retreat from egalitarian ideals and collective provision, and advocates instead minimal intervention in the economy and through the welfare system. Not surprisingly, free-market policies reward those who already hold the economic assets. This free-market approach took off in the UK in the late 1970s and, more importantly for global policy, the USA quickly followed suit. Facilitated by international financial institutions, global economic policy has required countries to open up their economies – and thus their labour markets and welfare systems – to greater foreign investment and control. It is a process fuelling the development of global commodities, like manufactured cigarettes and food products, which were originally developed for high-income consumers but now have their major markets in poorer countries. This form of globalization has high environmental and social costs, costs which disproportionately fall on the poorest countries and the poorest groups within countries. The costs are highest for their future children, a constituency with no voice in shaping the world into which they will be born.

The evidence suggests that the increasing worldwide dominance of the free-market system is both widening inequalities and restricting what national governments can do to contain them. This is particularly true for low- and middle-income countries seeking to develop and protect welfare institutions that distribute essential goods and services on a non-market basis. Nonetheless in high-income countries at least, policies continue to have a significant effect on the labour market and the welfare state, and thus on the scale of social inequality. Studies have focused on income inequalities for insight into the equity effects of government policies. They have found that the economies of high-income societies generate a highly unequal distribution of income. However, there continue to be differences in the extent to which national policies temper these market-generated inequalities. Some countries are much more effective than others in reducing poverty and equalizing incomes through their welfare systems.

What appears to distinguish them is their greater commitment to people's moral equality and to equality in what philosophers call basic freedoms. With this political commitment and the societal investments which follow from it, inequalities in people's lives can be and are being reduced. Without them, people's unequal lives are set to become increasingly unequal.

# Notes

## Introduction

1    The UK includes England, Wales, Scotland and Northern Ireland; Britain includes England, Wales and Scotland.

## Chapter 1

1    Daniels suggests a further reason for inferring that Rawls' vision of justice assumes that health determinants are fairly distributed. A society where there is uniformly good health for everyone would necessarily and inevitably be one where there is universally good access to health determinants (Daniels, 2002; Daniels *et al.*, 2004).

## Chapter 3

1    It should be noted that the concept of social capital has acquired a broader meaning in health research, and one largely detached from the operation of the class structure of high-income societies. For many health researchers, it is seen to describe the collective characteristics of groups – of neighbourhoods, regions and countries – including how much people interact with and trust each other, and their patterns of engagement in civic activities, like voting and voluntary work.

## Chapter 4

1    GNI is the term now used by the World Bank for gross national product (GNP).

## Chapter 10

1   The term 'critical period' is used for exposures which only have an effect during that time window: before and after it, there is no effect. An example is exposure to rubella *in utero*, with its adverse effects on foetal development limited to a relatively short time period in early pregnancy.

# References

Abberley, P. (1990) *Handicapped by Numbers: A Critique of the OPCS Disability Surveys*. Bristol: Bristol Polytechnic.

Adler, N.E. (2006) Overview of health disparities, in G.E. Thomson, F. Mitchell and M.B. Willaims (eds) *Examining the Health Disparities Research Plan of the National Institutes of Health*. Washington, DC: National Academies Press.

Ågren, G. (2003) *Sweden's New Public Health Policy*. Stockholm: National Institute for Public Health.

Aihie Sayer, A. and Cooper, C. (2004) A life course approach to biological ageing, in D.L. Kuh and Y. Ben-Shlomo (eds) *A Life Course Approach to Chronic Disease Epidemiology*, 2nd edn. Oxford: Oxford University Press.

Anand, S. and Peter, F. (2004) Introduction, in S. Anand, F. Peter and A. Sen (eds) *Public Health, Ethics and Equity*. Oxford: Oxford University Press.

Archer, L. and Francis, B. (2006) Challenging classes? Exploring the role of social class within the identities and achievement of Chinese pupils, *Sociology*, 40(1): 29–49.

Association of Public Health Observatories (APHO) (2005) *Indications of Public Health in the English Regions: 4. Ethnicity and Health*. www.apho.org.uk (accessed 3 February 2007).

Asthana, S. and Halliday, J. (2006) *What Works in Reducing Health Inequalities?* Bristol: Policy Press.

Atkinson, A.B. (1999) Income inequality in the UK, *Health Economics*, 8: 283–8.

Atkinson, A.B. (2002a) Seeking to explain the distribution of income, in J. Hills (ed.) *New Inequalities: The Changing Distribution of Income and Wealth in the United Kingdom*. Cambridge: Cambridge University Press.

Atkinson, A.B. (2005) Top incomes in the UK over the twentieth century, *Journal of the Royal Statistical Society*, 168(2): 325–43.

Atkinson, A.B., Rainwater, L. and Smeeding, T.M. (1995) *Income Distribution in OECD Countries*, Social Policy Studies No. 18. Paris: Organization for Economic Co-operation and Development.

Atkinson, T. (2002b) Is rising income inequality inevitable? in P. Townsend and D. Gordon (eds) *World Poverty: New Policies to Defeat an Old Enemy*. Bristol: Policy Press.

Bajekal, M., Blane, D., Grewal, I., Saffron, K. and Nazroo, J. (2004) Ethnic differences in influences on quality of life at older ages: a quantitative analysis, *Ageing and Society*, 24(5): 709–28.

Banks, J., Blundell, R. and Smith, J.P. (2003) Understanding differences in household financial wealth between the United States and Great Britain, *Journal of Human Resources*, 38(2): 241–79.

Banks, J., Marmot, M., Oldfield, Z. and Smith, J.P. (2006) Disease and disadvantage in the United States and in England, *Journal of the American Medical Association*, 295(17): 2037–45.

Barker, D.J.P. (1997) Fetal nutrition and cardiovascular disease in later life, *British Medical Bulletin*, 53(1): 96–108.

Barker, D.J.P. (1998) *Mothers, Babies and Health in Later Life*. Edinburgh: Churchill Livingstone.

Barn, R. with Ladino, C. and Brooke, R. (2006) *Parenting in Multi-racial Britain*. York: Joseph Rowntree Foundation.

Bartley, M. and Owen, C. (1996) Relation between socio-economic status, employment and health during economic change 1973–93, *British Medical Journal*, 313: 445–9.

Bartley, M., Calderwood, L., Jayaweera, H., Plewis, I. and Ward, K. (2005) Children's origins, in S. Dex and H. Joshi (eds) *Children of the 21st Century: From Birth to Nine Months*. Bristol: Policy Press.

Bartley, M., Sacker, A. and Schoon, I. (2002) Social and economic trajectories and women's health, in D. Kuh and R. Hardy (eds) *A Life Course Approach to Women's Health*. Oxford: Oxford University Press.

Belsky, J., Melhuish, E., Barnes, J., Leyland, A.H., Romanik, H. and the National Evalution of Sure Start Research Team (2006) Effects of Sure Start local programmes on children and families: early findings from a quasi-experimental, cross-sectional study, *British Medical Journal*, 332(7556): 1476–80.

Berridge, V. and Loughlin, K. (2005) Smoking and the new health education in Britain, 1950s–1970s, *American Journal of Public Health*, 95(6): 956–64.

Berthoud, R. (1998) *Incomes of Ethnic Minorities*, ISER Report. Essex: University of Essex.

Berthoud, R. and Blekesaune, M. (2006) *Persistent Employment Disadvantage, 1974 to 2003*, ISER working paper 2006–9. Essex: Institute of Social and Economic Research, University of Essex.

Bettie, J. (2000), Women without class, *Signs*, 26(1): 1–35.

Bhopal, R.S. (2002) *Concepts of Epidemiology*. Oxford: Oxford University Press.

Bickenbach, J.E., Chatterji, S., Badley, E.M. and Ustun, T.B. (1999) Models of disablement, universalism and the international classification of impairments, disabilities and handicaps, *Social Science and Medicine*, 48, 1173–87.

Birdsall, N. (2006) The world is not flat: inequality and injustice in our global economy. WIDER Annual Lecture 9. Helsinki, Finland, UNU World Institute for Development Economics Research (UNU-WIDER).

Blackburn, R.M. and Prandy, K. (1997) The reproduction of social inequality, *Sociology*, 31(3): 491–509.

Blakely, T., Woodward, A., Pearce, N. *et al.* (2002) Socio-economic factors and mortality among 25–64-year-olds from 1991–4: the New Zealand Census-Mortality Study, *New Zealand Medical Journal*, 115: 93–7.

Blanden, J., Goodman, A., Gregg, P. and Machin, S. (2001) *Changes in Intergenerational Mobility in Britain*. London: Centre for Economic Performance, London School of Economics.

Blanden, J., Gregg, P. and Machin, S. (2005) *Intergenerational Mobility in Europe and North America*. London: Centre for Economic Performance, London School of Economics.

Blane, D., Hart C.L., Smith, G.D. *et al.* (1996) Association of cardiovascular disease risk factors with socio-economic position during childhood and during adulthood, *British Medical Journal*, 313: 1434–8.

Blane, D., Smith, G.D. and Bartley, M. (1993) Social selection: what does it contribute to social class differences in health? *Sociology of Health and Illness*, 15(1): 1–15.

Bobak, M., Jha, P., Ngulen, S. and Jarvis, M. (2000) Poverty and smoking, in P. Jha and F. Chaloupka (eds) *Tobacco Control in Developing Countries*. Oxford: Oxford University Press.

Bommier, A. and Stecklov, G. (2002) Defining health inequality: why Rawls succeeds where social welfare theory fails, *Journal of Health Economics*, 21(3): 497–513.

Bottero, W. (2005) *Stratification: Social Division and Inequality*. London: Routledge.

Bourdieu, P. (1986) *Distinction*. Cambridge: Polity Press.

Bourdieu, P. (1990) *The Logic of Practice*. Cambridge: Polity Press.

Bowling, A. (2002) *Research Methods in Health: Investigating Health and Health Services*. Buckingham: Open University Press.

Boyce, W.T. and Keating, D.P. (2004) Should we intervene to improve fetal and infant growth? in D. Kuh and Y. Ben-Shlomo (eds) *A Life Course Approach to Chronic Disease Epidemiology*, 2nd edn. Oxford: Oxford University Press.

Bradshaw, J., Mayhew, E., Dex, S., Joshi, H. and Ward, K. (2005) Socio-economic origins of parents and child poverty, in S. Dex and H. Joshi (eds) *Children of the 21st Century: From Birth to Nine Months*. Bristol: Policy Press.

Braveman, P. (2006) Health disparities and health equity: concepts and measurement, *Annual Review of Public Health*, 27: 167–94.

Braveman, P. and Gruskin, S. (2003) Defining equity in health, *Journal of Epidemiology and Community Health*, 57: 254–8.

Braveman, P., Krieger, N. and Lynch, J. (2000) Health inequalities and social inequalities in health, *Bulletin of the World Health Organization*, 78(2): 232–4.

Braveman, P., Starfield, B. and Geiger, H.J. (2001) World Health Report 2000: how it removes equity from the agenda for public health monitoring and policy, *British Medical Journal*, 323: 678–80.

Breakwell, C. and Bajekal, M. (2006) Health expectancies in the UK and its constituent countries, 2001, *Health Statistics Quarterly*, 29: 18–25.

Breen, R. (2004) The comparative study of social mobility, in R. Breen (ed.) *Social Mobility in Europe*. Oxford: Oxford University Press.

Breen, R. and Goldthorpe, J.H. (2001) Class, mobility and merit: the experience of two British birth cohorts, *European Sociological Review*, 17(2): 81–101.

Breen, R. and Rottman, D.B. (1995) *Class Stratification: A Comparative Perspective*. Hemel Hempstead: Harvester Wheatsheaf.

Brennan, J. and Shah, T. (2003) *Access to What? Converting Educational Opportunity into Employment Opportunity*. London: Centre for Higher Education Research and Education.

Brewer, M., Goodman, A., Shaw, J. and Sibieta, L. (2006) *Poverty and Inequality in Britain*. London: Institute for Fiscal Studies, London.

Brimblecombe, N., Dorling, D. and Shaw, M. (2000) Migration and geographical inequalities in health in Britain, *Social Science and Medicine*, 50: 861–78.

Brock, A., Griffiths, C. and Rooney, C. (2006) The impact of introducing ICD-10 on analysis of respiratory mortality trends in England and Wales, *Health Statistics Quarterly*, 29: 9–17.

Bromley, C. (2003) Has Britain become immune to inequality? in A. Park, J. Curtice, K. Thomson, L. Jarvis and C. Bromley (eds) *British Social Attitudes: the Twentieth Report. Continuity and Change Over Two Decades*. London: Sage Publications.

Browne, J. and Stears, M. (2005) Capabilities, resources and systematic injustice: a case of gender inequality, *Politics, Philosophy and Economics*, 4(3): 355–73.

Brunner, E. and Marmot, M. (1999) Social organization, stress and health, in M. Marmot and R.G. Wilkinson (eds) *Social Determinants of Health*. Oxford: Oxford University Press.

Bunker, J. (2001) *Medicine Matters After All: Measuring the Benefits of Medical Care, a Healthy Lifestyle and a Just Social Environment*. London: Nuffield Trust.

Burchardt, T. (2005) *The Education and Employment of Disabled Young People: Frustrated Ambition*. Bristol: Policy Press.

Burghes, L. and Brown, M. (1995) *Single Lone Mothers: Problems, Prospects and Policies*. London: Family Policy Studies Centre and Joseph Rowntree Foundation.

Burström, B., Whitehead, M., Lindholm, C. *et al.* (2000) Inequality in the social consequences of illness: how well do people with long-term illness fare on the labour markets of Britain and Sweden? *International Journal of Health Services*, 30: 435–51.

Burton, L.M. (1990) Teenage childbearing as an alternative life-course strategy in multigeneration black families, *Human Nature*, 1(2): 123–43.

Bynner, J. (1999) New routes to employment: integration and exclusion, in W.R. Heinz (ed.) *From Education to Work: Cross-national Perspectives*. Cambridge: Cambridge University Press.

Bynner, J. and Pan, H. (2002) Changes in pathways to employment and family life?, in J. Bynner, P. Elias, A. McKnight, H. Pan and G. Pierre (eds) *Young People's Changing Routes to Independence*. York: Joseph Rowntree Foundation.

Byrne, B. (2006) In search of a 'good mix': race, class, gender and practices of mothering, *Sociology*, 40(6): 1001–17.

Calderwood, L., Kiernan, K., Joshi, H., Smith, K. and Ward, K. (2005) Parenthood and parenting, in S. Dex and H. Joshi (eds) *Children of the 21st Century*. Bristol: Policy Press.

Callender, C. and Wilkinson, D. (2004) *2002–3 Student Income and Expenditure Survey*, research report RR487. London: Department for Education and Skills.

Campbell, D. (2006) They've got it all, Observer, 6th August: 3.

Campbell, J. and Oliver, M. (1996) *Disability Politics: Understanding Our Past, Changing Our Future*. London: Routledge.

Carolina, M.S. and Gustavo, L.F. (2003) Epidemiological transition: model or illusion? A look at the problem of health in Mexico, *Social Science & Medicine*, 57: 539–50.

Cavelaars, A.E., Kunst, A.E. and Mackenbach, J.P. (1997) Socio-economic differences in risk factors for morbidity and mortality in the European Community, *Journal of Health Psychology*, 2(3): 353–72.

Cavelaars, A.E., Kunst A.E., Geurts J.J. et al. (2000) Educational differences in smoking: international comparison. *British Medical Journal*, 320(7242): 1102–7.

Charlesworth, S.J. (2000) *A Phenomenology of Working Class Experience*. Cambridge: Cambridge University Press.

Charlton, J. and Murphy, M. (1997) Trends in causes of mortality: 1841–1994 – an overview, in Office for National Statistics (ed.) *The Health of Adult Britain 1841–1994*. London: The Stationery Office.

Chopra, M. and Darnton-Hill, I. (2004) Tobacco and obesity epidemics: not so different after all? *British Medical Journal*, 328: 1558–60.

Clark, T.N. and Lipset, S.M. (1991) Are social classes dying? *International Sociology*, 6(4): 397–410.

Commission on Health Research for Development (CHRD) (1990) *Health Research: Essential Link to Equity in Development*. Oxford: Oxford University Press.

Commission on Social Determinants of Health (CSDH) (2005) *Action on Social Determinants of Health: Learning from Previous Experiences*, background paper prepared for the Commission on Social Determinants of Health, WHO. Geneva: WHO.

Commission on Social Determinants of Health (CSDH) (2006) *Commission on Social Determinants of Health*, ref. WHO/EIP/EQH/01/2006. WHO. Geneva: WHO.

Corlynon, J. and McGuire, C. (1999) *Pregnancy and Parenthood: The Views and Experiences of Young People in Public Care*. London: National Children's Bureau.

Cornia, G.A. (2001) Globalization and health: results and options, *Bulletin of the World Health Organization*, 79(9): 834–41.

Crompton, R. (1993) *Class and Stratification: An Introduction to Current Debates*. Cambridge: Polity Press.

Crompton, R., Brockmann, M. and Lyonette, C. (2005) Attitudes, women's employment and the domestic division of labour: a cross-national analysis in two waves. *Work, Employment and Society*, 19(2): 213–33.

Dahlgren, G. and Whitehead, M. (1991) *Policies and Strategies to Promote Equity in Health*. Stockholm: Institute for Future Studies.

Dahlgren, G. and Whitehead, M. (1993) *Tackling Inequalities in Health: What Can We Learn From What Has Been Tried?* working paper prepared for the King's Fund International Seminar on Tackling Inequalities in Health, September, Ditchley Park, Oxfordshire. London: King's Fund.

Dahlgren, G. and Whitehead, M. (2006) *Levelling Up II: A Discussion Paper on European Strategies to Tackle Social Inequities in Health.* Copenhagen: WHO.

Dalziel, P. (2002) New Zealand's economic reforms: an assessment, *Review of Political Economy*, 14(1): 31–46.

Daniels, N. (2002) Democratic equality: Rawls' complex egalitarianism, in S. Freeman (ed.) *The Cambridge Companion to Rawls.* Cambridge: Cambridge University Press.

Daniels, N., Kennedy, B.P. and Kawachi, I. (1999) Why justice is good for our health: the social determinants of health inequalities, *Daedalus*, 128(4): 215–51.

Daniels, N., Kennedy, B. and Kawachi, I. (2004) Health and inequality or why justice is good for our health, in S. Anand, F. Peter and A. Sen (eds) *Public Health, Ethics and Society.* Oxford: Oxford University Press.

Davey Smith, G. (1997) Socio-economic differentials, in D.L. Kuh and Y. Ben-Shlomo (eds) *A Life Course Approach to Chronic Disease Epidemiology.* Oxford: Oxford University Press.

Davey Smith, G., Gunnell, D. and Ben-Shlomo, Y. (2001) Life course approaches to socio-economic differentials in cause-specific adult mortality, in D. Leon and G. Walt (eds) *Poverty, Inequality and Health.* Oxford: Oxford University Press.

Davey Smith, G., Hart C., Blane, D., Gillis, C. and Hawthorne, V. (1997) Lifetime socio-economic position and mortality: prospective observational study, *British Medical Journal*, 314: 547–52.

De Beyer, J., Lovelace, C. and Yürekli, A. (2001) Poverty and tobacco, *Tobacco Control*, 10: 210–11.

Deacon, A. and Bradshaw, J. (1983) *Reserved for the Poor: The Means Test in British Social Policy.* Oxford: Basil Blackwell and Martin Robertson.

Deaton, A. (2003) Health, inequality and economic development, *Journal of Economic Literature*, 41(1): 113–15 (113–58 in e-journal).

Deaton, A. (2006) *Global Patterns of Income and Health: Facts, Interpretations and Policies*, WIDER Annual Lecture, September, Helsinki, Finland.

Demakakos, P., Hacker, E. and Gjonça, E. (2006) Perceptions of ageing, in J. Banks, E. Breeze, C. Lessof and J. Nazroo (eds) *Retirement, Health and Relationships of the Older Population in England: The 2004 English Longitudinal Study of Ageing (Wave 2).* London: Institute of Fiscal Studies.

Department for Education and Skills (DfES) (2003) *Youth Cohort Study: The Activities and Experiences of 18-year-olds: England and Wales 2002*, SFR 04/2003. London: Department for Education and Skills.

Department for Education and Skills (DfES) (2006) *National Curriculum Assessment, GCSE and Equivalent Attainment and Post-16 Attainment by Pupil Characteristics in England, 2005*, ref. ID SFR091/2006. London: Department for Education and Skills.

Department of Health (DoH) (2001) *Tackling Health Inequalities: Consultation on a Plan for Delivery*. London: Department of Health.

Department of Health (DoH) (2002) *Tackling Health Inequalities: 2002 Cross-Cutting Review*. London: Department of Health.

Department of Health (DoH) (2005) *Tackling Health Inequalities: Status Report on the Programme for Action*. London: Department of Health.

Department of Health (DoH) (2006) *Tackling Health Inequalities: Status Report on the Programme for Action – 2006 Update of Headline Indicators*. London: Department of Health.

Department of Health and Children (DHC) (2001) *Quality and Fairness: A Health System for You*. Dublin: The Stationery Office.

Department of Health and Human Services (DHHS) (2000) *Healthy People 2010, Volume 1*. www.healthypeople.gov/document (accessed 3 February 2007).

Department of Health, Social Services and Public Safety (DHSSPS) (2000) *Investing in Health: A Consultation Paper*. Belfast: DHSSPS.

Devis, T. and Rooney, C. (1999) Death certification and the epidemiologist, *Health Statistics Quarterly*, 1: 21–33.

Dezateux, C., Bedford, H., Cole, T. *et al*. (2004) Babies' health and development, in S. Dex and H. Joshi (eds) *Millennium Cohort Study First Survey: A User's Guide to Initial Findings*. London: Centre for Longitudinal Studies, Institute of Education, University of London.

Dickens, R. (2000) Caught in a trap? Wage mobility in Great Britain: 1975–94, *Economica*, 67: 477–97.

Diderichsen, F. (1998) Understanding equity in populations, in E. Arve-Pares (ed.) *Promoting Research on Inequality in Health*. Stockholm: Swedish Council for Social Research.

Diderichsen, F., Evans, T. and Whitehead, M. (2001) The social basis of disparities in health, in T. Evans, M. Whitehead, F. Diderichsen, A. Bhuiya and M. Wirth (eds) *Challenging Inequities in Health: from Ethics to Action*. Oxford: Oxford University Press.

Doll, R. and Hill, A.B. (1950) Smoking and carcinoma of the lung. Preliminary report, *British Medical Journal*, ii: 739–48C.

Doll. R., Darby, S. and Whitley, E. (1997) Trends in mortality from smoking-related diseases, in Office for National Statistics (ed.) *The Health of Adult Britain 1841–1994*. London: The Stationery Office.

Doran, T. and Whitehead, M. (2004) Do social policies and political context matter for health in the United Kingdom? in V. Navarro (ed.) *The Political and Social Contexts of Health*. New York, NY: Baywood Publishing.

Dorling, D., Shaw, M. and Davey Smith, G. (2006) Global inequality of life expectancy due to AIDS, *British Medical Journal*, 332: 662–4.

Dorsett, R. and Marsh, A. (1998) *The Health Trap: Poverty, Smoking and Lone Parenthood*. London: Policy Studies Institute.

Douglas, J.W.B. and Blomfield, J.M. (1958) *Children Under Five*. London: George Allen and Unwin.

Doyal, L. with Pennell, I. (1979) *The Political Economy of Health*. London: Pluto Press.

Drever, F. and Bunting, J. (1997) Patterns and trends in male mortality, in F. Drever and M. Whitehead (eds) *Health Inequalities*. London: Office for National Statistics.

Drever, F. and Whitehead, M. (eds) (1997) *Health Inequalities*. London: Office for National Statistics.

Drever, F., Whitehead, M. and Rodin, M. (1996) Current patterns and trends in male mortality by social class (based on occupation), *Population Trends*, 86: 15–20.

Drewnowski, A. and Popkin, B.M. (1997) The nutrition transition: new trends in the global diet, *Nutrition Reviews*, 55(2): 31–43.

Drèze, J. and Sen, A. (1989) *Hunger and Public Action*. Oxford: Clarendon Press.

Efroymson, D., Ahmed, S., Townsend, J. *et al.* (2001) Hungry for tobacco: an analysis of the economic impact of tobacco consumption on the poor in Bangladesh, *Tobacco Control*, 10(3): 212–17.

Egerton, M. and Savage, M. (2000) Age stratification and class formation: a longitudinal study of the social mobility of young men and women, 1971–91, *Work, Employment and Society*, 14(1): 23–49.

Elias, P. and Purcell, K. (2004) *The Earnings of Graduates in Their Early Careers*, research paper no. 5. Warwick: Institute for Employment Research, University of Warwick.

Elo, I.R. and Preston, S.H. (1996) Educational differentials in mortality: United States, 1979–85, *Social Science and Medicine*, 42(1): 47–57.

Emerson, E., Graham, H. and Hatton, C. (2006) Household income and health status in children and adolescents in Britain, *European Journal of Public Health*, 16(4): 354–60.

Emerson, E., Malam, S., Spencer, K. and Davies, I. (2005) *Adults with Learning Disabilities in England 2003–4*. Leeds: Health and Social Care Information Centre.

Erens, B., McManus, S., Field, J., Korovessis, C., Johnson, A.M. and Fenton, K.A. (2003) *National Survey of Sexual Attitudes and Lifestyles II: Reference Tables and Summary*. London: National Centre for Social Research.

Erens, B., Primatesta, P. and Prior, G. (eds) (2001) *Health Survey for England 1999: The Health of Minority Ethnic Groups*. London: The Stationery Office.

Erikson, R. and Goldthorpe, J.H. (2002) Intergenerational inequality: a sociological perspective, *Journal of Economic Perspectives*, 16(3): 31–44.

Ermisch, J. (2003) *Does a 'Teen-birth' have Longer-term Impacts on the Mother?* working paper 2003–32. Colchester: Institute for Social and Economic Research, University of Essex.

Ermisch, J., Francesconi, M. and Siedler, T. (2006) Intergenerational mobility and marital sorting, *The Economic Journal*, 116: 659–79.

Esping-Andersen, G. (1990) *The Three Worlds of Welfare Capitalism*. Princeton, NJ: Princeton University Press.

Esping-Andersen, G. (1993) Post-industrial class structures: an analytical framework, in G. Esping-Andersen (ed.) *Changing Classes: Stratification and Social Mobility in Post-Industrial Societies*. London: Sage.

Esping-Andersen, G. (2004) Unequal opportunities and the mechanism of social inheritance, in M. Corak (ed.) *Generational Income Mobility in North America and Europe*. Cambridge: Cambridge University Press.

Evandrou, M. and Falkingham, J. (1995) Gender, lone parenthood and lifetime income, in J. Falkingham and J. Hills (eds) *The Dynamic of Welfare: The Welfare State and the Life Cycle*. Hemel Hemsptead: Prentice Hall/Harvester Wheatsheaf.

Evans, E.J. (ed.) (1978) *Social Policy 1830–1914*. London: Routledge and Kegan Paul.

Evans, R.G. and Stoddart, G.L. (1990) Producing health, consuming health care, *Social Science and Medicine*, 31(12): 1347–63.

Evans, T., Whitehead, M., Diderichsen, F., Bhuiya, A. and Wirth, M. (eds) (2001) *Challenging Inequities in Health: from Ethics to Action*. Oxford: Oxford University Press.

Falkingham, J. and Hills, J. (1995a) The effects of the welfare state over the life cycle, in J. Falkingham and J. Hills (eds) *The Dynamic of Welfare: The Welfare State and the Life Cycle*. Hemel Hempstead: Prentice Hall/Harvester Wheatsheaf.

Falkingham, J. and Hills, J. (1995b) Lifetime incomes and the welfare state, in J. Falkingham and J. Hills (eds) *The Dynamic of Welfare: The Welfare State and the Life Cycle*. Hemel Hempstead: Prentice Hall/Harvester Wheatsheaf.

Farr, W. (1885) Life and death in England, in N.A. Humphreys (ed.) *Vital Statistics: A Memorial Volume of Selections from the Reports and Writings of William Farr*. London: Sanitory Institute of Great Britain. Reprinted in *Bulletin of the World Health Organization*, 2000, 78(1): 88–96.

Ferguson, J., Bauld, L., Chesterman, J. and Judge, K. (2005) The English smoking treatment services: one-year outcomes, *Addiction*, 100 (Suppl. 2): 59–69.

Fergusson, R. (2004), Discourses of exclusion: reconceptualizing participation among young people, *Journal of Social Policy*, 33(2): 289–320.

Fernando, D. (2000) Health care systems in transition III. Sri Lanka, Part 1: an overview of Sri Lanka's health care system, *Journal of Public Health Medicine*, 22(1): 14–20.

Ferri, E. and Smith, K. (2003) Partnerships and parenthood, in E. Ferri, J. Bynner and M. Wadsworth (eds) *Changing Britain, Changing Lives*. London: Bedford Way Papers.

Fisher, G.M. (1992) The development and history of the poverty thresholds, *Social Security Bulletin*, 55(4): 3–14.

Fox, K. (2004) *Watching the English: The Hidden Rules of English Behaviour*. London: Hodder.

Frankenburg, R. (1997) Local whitenesses, localizing whiteness, in R. Frankenburg (ed.) *Displacing Whiteness: Essays in Social and Cultural Criticism*. Durham, NC: Duke University Press.

Freeman, S. (ed.) (2002) *The Cambridge Companion to Rawls*. Cambridge: Cambridge University Press.

Fritzell, J. (2001) Still different? Income distribution in the Nordic countries in the European context, in M. Kautto, J. Fritzell, B. Hvinden, J. Kvist and H. Uusitalo (eds) *Nordic Welfare States in the European Context*. London: Routledge.

Fritzell, J. and Lundberg, O. (2006) Health inequalities, welfare and resources, in J. Fritzell and O. Lundberg (eds) *Health Inequalities and Welfare Resources*. Bristol: Policy Press.

Furlong, A. and Cartmel, F. (2005) *Graduates from Disadvantaged Families*. York: Joseph Rowntree Foundation.

Gajalakshmi, C.K., Jha, P., Ranson, K. and Nguyen, S. (2000) Global patterns of smoking and smoking-attributable mortality, in P. Jha and F. Chaloupka (eds) *Tobacco Control in Developing Countries*. Oxford: Oxford University Press.

Galobardes, B., Lynch, J.W. and Davey Smith, G. (2004) Childhood socio-economic circumstances and cause-specific mortality in adulthood: systematic review and interpretation, *Epidemiologic Reviews*, 26: 7–21.

Gangl, M., Muller, W. and Raffe, D. (2004) Conclusions: explaining cross-national differences in school-to-work transitions, in M. Gangl, W. Muller and D. Raffe (eds) *Transitions from Education to Work in Europe: The Integration of Youth into EU Labour Markets*. Oxford: Oxford University Press.

Gans, H.J. (2005) Race as class, *Contexts*, 4(4): 17–21.

Gimenez, M.E. (2006) With a little class: a critique of identity politics, *Ethnicities*, 6(3): 423–39.

Ginsberg, N. (1993) Sweden: the social democratic case, in A. Cochrane and J. Clarke (eds) *Comparing Welfare States: Britain in International Context*. Milton Keynes: The Open University.

Glass, D.V. (ed.) (1954) *Social Mobility in Britain*. London: Routledge and Kegan Paul.

Glyn, A. (2006) *Capitalism Unleashed: Finance, Globalization and Welfare*. Oxford: Oxford University Press.

Goesling, B. and Firebaugh, G. (2004) The trend in international health inequality, *Population and Development Review*, 30(1): 131–6.

Goldthorpe, J.H. and Mills, C. (2004) Trends in intergenerational class mobility in Britain in the late twentieth century, in R. Breen (ed.) *Social Mobility in Europe*. Oxford: Oxford University Press.

Goodman, A. and Shepherd, P. (2002) *Inequality and Living Standards in Great Britain: Some Facts*. London: Institute for Fiscal Studies.

Goodman, J. (1993) *Tobacco in History*. London: Routledge.

Graham, H. (1993) *When Life's a Drag: Women, Smoking and Disadvantage*. London: HMSO.

Graham, H. (1996) Smoking prevalence among women in the European Community 1950–90, *Social Science and Medicine*, 3: 242–7.

Graham, H. and Der, G. (1999) Influences on women's smoking status: the contribution of socio-economic status in adolescence and adulthood, *European Journal of Public Health*, 9: 137–41.

Graham, H., Francis, B., Inskip, H., Harman, J. and SWS Study Team (2006a) Socio-economic lifecourse influences on women's smoking status in early adulthood, *Journal of Epidemiology and Community Health*, 60: 228–33.

Graham, H., Inskip, H. Francis, B. and Harman, J. (2006b) Pathways of disadvantage and smoking careers: evidence and policy implications, *Journal of Epidemiology and Community Health*, 60(Suppl 11): ii7–ii12.

Green, A.E. and Owen, D. (1998) *Where Are the Jobless?* Bristol: Polity Press.

Green, F. (1999) Training the workers, in P. Gregg and J. Wadsworth (eds) *The State of Working Britain*. Manchester: Manchester University Press.

Green, H., McGinnity, A., Meltzer, H. *et al.* (2005) *Mental Health of Children and Young People in Great Britain, 2004*. London: Office for National Statistics.

Gregg, P. and Wadsworth, J. (1996) More work in fewer households, in J. Hills (ed.) *New Inequalities: The Changing Distribution of Income and Wealth in the United Kingdom*. Cambridge, Cambridge University Press.

Griffiths, C. and Brock, A. (2003) Twentieth century mortality trends in England and Wales, *Health Statistics Quarterly*, 18: 5–17.

Grundy, E. and Glaser, K. (2000) Socio-demographic differences in the onset and progression of disability in early old age: a longitudinal study, *Age and Ageing*, 29: 149–57.

Gubéran, E. and Usel, M. (1998) Permanent work incapacity, mortality and survival without work incapacity among occupations and social classes: a cohort study of ageing men in Geneva, *International Journal of Epidemiology*, 27: 1026–32.

Guralnik, J., Butterworth, S., Wadsworth, M.E.J. and Kuh, D. (2006) Childhood socio-economic status predicts physical functioning half a century later, *Journal of Gerontology Series A: Biological Sciences and Medical Sciences*, 61: 694–701.

Gwatkin, D.R., Rustein, S., Johnson, K., Parde, R.P. and Wagstaff, A. (2000) *India: Socio-economic Differences in Health, Nutrition and Population*. Washington, DC: World Bank.

Halfon, N. and Hochstein, M. (2002) Life course health development: an integrated framework for developing health, policy and research, *The Milbank Quarterly*, 80(3): 433–79.

Hammond, R.J. (1951) *Food*, History of the Second World War, United Kingdom Civil Series. London: HM Stationery Office.

Harper, S., Lynch, J., Wan-Ling, H. *et al.* (2002) Life course socio-economic conditions and adult psychosocial functioning, *International Journal of Epidemiology*, 31: 395–403.

Harris, T. (2000) The effects of taxes and benefits on household income, 1998–9, *Economic Trends*, 557: 45–83.

Harrison, E. (2006) Social class in Britain, *ISER Newsletter*, Summer: 1–2. Colchester: Institute for Social and Economic Research, University of Essex.

Health Statistics Quarterly (HSQ) (2006a) Report: death registrations in England and Wales: 2005, causes, *Health Statistics Quarterly*, 30: 46–55.

Health Statistics Quarterly (HSQ) (2006b) Report: health expectancies in the UK, 2002, *Health Statistics Quarterly*, 29: 59–62.

Heath, A.F. and Ridge, J.M. (1983) Social mobility of ethnic minorities, *Journal of Biosocial Science*, 8: 169–84.

Hertzman, C. (1999) Population health and human development, in C. Hertzman and D.P. Keating (eds) *Developmental Health and the Wealth of Nation*. London: Guildford Press.

Hertzman, C. (2001) Population health and child development: a view from Canada, in J.A. Auerbach and B. Krimgold (eds) *Income, Socio-economic Status and Health: Exploring the Relationships*. London: National Policy Association.

Hickman, M.J. (2005) Ruling an empire, governing a multinational state, in G.C. Loury, T. Modood and S.M. Teles (eds) *Ethnicity, Social Mobility and Public Policy*. Cambridge: Cambridge University Press.

Hicks, J. and Allen, G. (1999) *A Century of Change: Trends in UK Statistics since 1900*, research paper 99/111. London: Social and General Statistics Section, House of Commons Library. www.parliament.uk/commons/lib/research/rp99/rp99–111.pdf (accessed on 14 December 2006).

Hills, J. (2004) *Inequality and the State*. Oxford: Oxford University Press.

Hilton, M. (2000) *Smoking in British Popular Culture 1800–2000*. Manchester: Manchester University Press.

Hinde, S. and Dixon, J. (2004) Changing the obesogenic environment: insights from a cultural economy of car reliance, *Transportation Research Part D*, 10: 31–53.

Hobcraft, J. and Kiernan, K. (2001) Childhood poverty, early motherhood and adult social exclusion, *British Journal of Sociology*, 52(3): 495–517.

Holtzman, N.A. (2002) Genetics and social class, *Journal of Epidemiology and Community Health*, 56: 529–35.

Homedes, N. and Ugalde, A. (2005) Why neoliberal reforms have failed Latin America, *Health Policy*, 71: 83–96.

House, J.S. and Williams, D.R. (2000) Understanding and explaining socio-economic and racial/ethnic disparities in health, in B.D. Smedley and S.L. Syme (eds) *Promoting Health: Intervention Strategies from Social and Behavioural Health*. Washington, DC: National Academy Press.

Huisman, M., Kunst, A.E. and Mackenbach, J.P. (2005) Educational inequalities in smoking among men and women aged 16 years and older in 11 European countries, *Tobacco Control*, 14: 106–13.

Humpage, L. and Fleras, A. (2001) Intersecting discourses: closing the gaps, social justice and the Treaty of Waitangi, *Social Policy of New Zealand*, 16: 37–53.

Idler, E.L. and Benyamini, Y. (1997) Self-rated health and mortality: a review of 27 community studies, *Journal of Health and Social Behaviour*, 38: 21–37.

Illich, I. (1975) *Medical Nemesis: The Expropriation of Health*. London: Caldar and Boyers.

Inskip, H.M., Godfrey, K.M., Robinson, S.M. *et al.* (2006) Cohort profile: the Southampton Women's Survey, *International Journal of Epidemiology*, 35: 42–8.

Institute for Fiscal Studies (IFS) website, *Inequality, Poverty and Well-being Spreadsheet*. www.ifs.org.uk/projects_research.php?heading_id=8_ (accessed 18 January 2007).

Jacobs, J.A. and Gerson, K. (2004) *The Time Divide: Work, Family and Gender Inequality*. Cambridge, MA: Harvard University Press.

Jarvis, S. and Jenkins, S.P. (1998) Marital dissolution and income change, in R. Ford and J. Millar (eds) *Private Lives and Public Responses*. London: Policy Studies Institute.

Jebb, S.A., Lang, R. and Penrose, A. (2003) Improving communication to tackle obesity, *Proceedings of the Nutrition Society*, 62: 577–81.

Jefferis, B. J., Graham, H., Manor, O. and Power, C. (2003) Level of cigarette smoking and socio-economic circumstances in adolescence: how do they affect adult smoking? *Addiction*, 98: 1765–72.

Jefferis, B., Power, C. and Hertzman, C. (2002) Birthweight, childhood socio-economic environment and cognitive development in the 1958 British birth cohort, *British Medical Journal*, 325: 305–8.

Jefferis, B.J., Power, C., Graham, H. and Manor, O. (2004a) Changing social gradients in cigarette smoking and cessation over two decades of adult follow- up in a British birth cohort, *Journal of Public Health Medicine*, 26(1): 13–18.

Jefferis, J.M.H., Power, C., Graham, H. and Manor, O. (2004b) Effects of childhood socio-economic circumstances on persistent smoking. *American Journal of Public Health*, 94: 279–85.

Jones, C. (1991) Birth statistics 1990, *Population Trends*, 65: 9–15.

Jones, F. (2005) The effects of taxes and benefits on household income, 2003–4, *Economic Trends*, 620: 15–60.

Joseph, K. (1977) *Monetarism Is Not Enough*. London: Centre for Policy Studies.

Joshi, H. (2002) Production, reproduction and education: women, children and work in a British perspective, *Population and Development Review*, 28(3): 445–74.

Jotangia, D., Moody, A., Stamatakis, E. and Wardle, H. (2005) *Obesity among Children under 11*. London: Office for National Statistics.

Judge, K., Platt, S., Costongs, C. and Jurczak, K. (2005) *Health Inequalities: A Challenge for Europe*, an independent expert report commissioned by and published under the auspices of the UK Presidency of the EU. London: Central Office of Information.

Keating, D. and Hertzman, C. (1999) *Developmental Health and the Wealth of Nations*. New York, NY: Guilford Press.

Kiernan, K. and Pickett, K.E. (2006) Marital status disparities in maternal smoking during pregnancy, breastfeeding and maternal depression, *Social Science and Medicine*, 63: 335–46.

Kiernan, K.E. (2004) Unmarried cohabitation and parenthood in Britain and Europe, *Journal of Law and Policy*, 26(1): 33–5.

Kiernan, K.E. and Eldridge, S.M. (1987) Age at marriage: inter and intra cohort variation, *British Journal of Sociology*, 38(1): 44–65.

King, A. (2000) *The New Zealand Health Strategy*.Wellington: Ministry of Health.

Kinra, S., Nelder, R. and Lewendon, G. (2005) Deprivation and childhood obesity: a cross-sectional study of 20,973 in Plymouth, United Kingdom, *Journal of Epidemiology and Community Health*, 54: 456–60.

Kramer, M.S., Séguin, L., Lydon, J. and Goulet, L. (2000) Socio-economic disparities in pregnancy outcome: why do the poor fare so badly? *Paediatric and Perinatal Epidemiology*, 14: 194–210.

Krieger, N. (1994) Epidemiology and the web of causation: has anyone seen the spider? *Social Science and Medicine*, 39: 887–903.

Krieger, N. (1997) Measuring social class in US public health research, *American Review of Public Health*, 18: 341–78.

Krieger, N. (2000) Discrimination and health, in L.F. Berkman and I. Kawachi (eds) *Social Epidemiology*. Oxford: Oxford University Press.

Krieger, N. (2001) A glossary for social epidemiology, *Journal of Epidemiology and Community Health*, 55: 693–700.

Kuh, D. and Ben-Shlomo, Y. (eds) (2004) *A Life Course Approach to Chronic Disease Epidemiology*. Oxford: Oxford University Press.

Kuh, D., Ben-Shlomo, Y., Lynch, J., Hallqvist, J. and Power, C. (2003) Glossary: life course epidemiology, *Journal of Epidemiology and Community Health*, 57: 778–83.

Kuh, D., Hardy, R., Langenberg, C., Richards, M. and Wadsworth, M.E. (2002) Mortality in adults aged 26–54 years related to socio-economic conditions in childhood and adulthood: post-war birth cohort study, *British Medical Journal*, 325(7372): 1076–80.

Kuh, D., Power, C., Blane, D. and Bartley, M. (2004) Socio-economic pathways between childhood and adult health, in D.L. Kuh and Y. Ben-Shlomo (eds) *A Life Course Approach to Chronic Disease Epidemiology*, 2nd edn. Oxford: Oxford University Press.

Kunst, A.E. Bos, V., Lahelma, E. *et al.* (2005) Trends in socio-economic inequalities in self-assessed health in ten European countries, *International Journal of Epidemiology*, 34: 295–305.

Kunst, A.E., Groenhof, F. and Mackenbach, J.P. and the EU Working Group on Socio-economic Inequalities in Health (1998) Mortality by occupational class among men 30–64 years in 11 European countries, *Social Science and Medicine*, 46(11): 1459–76.

Kutty, V.R. (2001) Reforms and their relevance: the Kerala experience, in I. Qadeer, K. Sen and K.R. Nayar (eds) *Public Health and the Poverty of Reforms*. New Delhi: Sage.

Kymlicka, W. (2002) *Contemporary Political Philosophy: An Introduction*. Oxford: Oxford University Press.

Labonte, R. and Schrecker, T. (2005) A global health equity agenda for the G8 summit, *British Medical Journal*, 330: 533–6.

Labonte, R. and Schrecker, T. (2006) *Globalization and Social Determinants of Health: Analytic and Strategic Review Paper*. Ontario, Ottawa: Institute of Population Health.

Lahelma, E., Keskimäki, I. and Rahkonen, O. (2002) Income maintenance policies: the example of Finland, in J.P. Mackenbach and M.J. Bakker (eds) *Reducing Health Inequalities: A European Perspective*. London: Routledge.

Lalonde, M. (1974) *A New Perspective on the Health of Canadians: A Working Document*. Ottawa: Minister of Supply and Services Canada.

Lancet Editorial (1843), *The Lancet*, 1040: 657–61.

Lareau, A. (2003) *Unequal Childhoods: Class, Race and Family Life*. London: University of California Press.

Lawlor, D.A., Ben-Shlomo, Y. and Leon, D.A. (2004) Pre-adult influences on cardiovascular disease, in D.L. Kuh and Y. Ben-Shlomo (eds) *A Life Course Approach to Chronic Disease Epidemiology*, 2nd edn. Oxford: Oxford University Press.

Le Grand, J. (1982) *The Strategy of Equality: Redistribution and the Social Services*. London: George Allen and Unwin.

Le Grand, J. (1991) *Equity and Choice*. London: HarperCollins.

Leatherman, T.L. and Goodman, A. (2005) Coca-colonization of diets in the Yucatan, *Social Science and Medicine*, 61: 833–46.

Lee, P.N. (1975) *Tobacco Consumption in Various Countries*. London: Tobacco Research Council.

Leventhal, T. and Brooks-Gunn, J. (2000) The neighbourhoods they live in: the effects of neighbourhood residence on child and adolescent outcomes, *Psychological Bulletin*, 126(2): 309–37.

Lewis, J. (1986) *What Price Community Medicine? The Philosophy, Practice and Politics of Public Health since 1919*. Brighton: Wheatsheaf Books.

Lindholm, C., Burström, B. and Diderichsen, F. (2002) Class differences in the social consequences of illness? *Journal of Epidemiology and Community Health*, 56: 188–92.

Link, B.G. and Phelan, J. (1995) Social conditions as fundamental causes of disease, *Journal of Health and Social Behaviour*, extra issue: 80–94.

Lopez, A.D., Mathers, C.D., Ezzati, M., Jamison, D.T. and Murray, C.J.L. (2006) *Global Burden of Disease and Risk Factors*. Oxford: Oxford University Press and World Bank.

Lopez, A.D., Salomon, J., Ahmad, O., Murray, C.J.L. and Mafat, D. (2001) *Life Tables for 191 Countries: Data, Methods and Results*, discussion paper no 9. Geneva: World Health Organization.

Loury, G.C., Modood, T. and Teles, S.M. (2005) Introduction, in G.C. Loury, T. Modood and S.M. Teles (eds) *Ethnicity, Social Mobility and Public Policy.* Cambridge: Cambridge University Press.

Lundberg, O. and Lahelma, E. (2001) Nordic health inequalities in the European context, in M. Kautto, J. Fritzell, B. Hvinden, J. Kvist and H. Uusitalo (eds) *Nordic Welfare States in the European Context.* London: Routledge.

Lynch, J.W., Kaplan, G.A. and Shema, S.J. (1997) Cumulative impact of sustained economic hardship on physical, cognitive, psychological and social functioning, *New England Journal of Medicine*, 337(26): 1889–95.

Machin, S. (2003) Unto them that hath . . ., *CentrePiece*, 8(1): 5–9.

Machin, S. and Vignoles, A. (2004) Educational inequality: the widening socio-economic gap, *Fiscal Studies*, 25(2): 107–28.

Mackenbach, J.P. (1996) The contribution of medical care to mortality decline: McKeown revisited, *Journal of Clinical Epidemiology*, 49(11): 1207–13.

Mackenbach, J.P. (2005a) *Health Inequalities: Europe in Profile*, an independent expert report commissioned by and published under the auspices of the UK Presidency of the EU, Erasmus MC University Medical Center, Rotterdam.

Mackenbach, J.P. (2005b) Genetics and health inequalities: hypotheses and controversies, *Journal of Epidemiology and Community Health*, 59: 268–73.

Mackenbach, J.P. and Bakker, M.J. for the European Network on Interventions and Policies to Reduce Inequalities in Health (2003) Tackling socio-economic inequalities in health: analysis of European experiences, *The Lancet*, 362: 1409–14.

Mackenbach, J.P., Bakker, M.J., Kunst, A.E. and Diderichsen, F. (2002) Socio-economic inequalities in Europe: an overview, in J.P. Mackenbach and M.J. Bakker (eds) *Reducing Health Inequalities: A European Perspective.* London: Routledge.

Mackenbach, J.P., Looman, C.W., Kunst, A.E., Habbema, J.D. and van der Maas, P.J. (1988) Post-1950 mortality trends and medical care: gains in life expectancy due to declines in mortality from conditions amenable to medical intervention in The Netherlands, *Social Science and Medicine*, 27: 889–94.

Mackenbach, J.P., van de Mheen, H. and Stronks, K. (1994) A prospective cohort study investigating the explanation of socio-economic inequalities in health in The Netherlands, *Social Science and Medicine*, 38(2): 299–308.

Magnuson, K.A. and Duncan, G.J. (2002) Parents in poverty, in M.H. Bornstein (ed.) *Handbook of Parenting, Volume 4 Social Conditions and Parenting.* London: Lawrence Erlbaum Associates.

Manning, A. (2006) The gender pay gap, *Centre Piece*, 11(1): 13–16.

Manor, O., Matthews, S. and Power, C. (1997) Comparing measures of health inequality, *Social Science and Medicine*, 45(5): 761–71.

Marmot, M., Banks, J., Blundell, R., Lessof, C. and Nazroo, J. (2003) Introduction, in M. Marmot, J. Banks, R. Blundell, C. Lessof, and J. Nazroo (eds) *Health, Wealth and Lifestyles of the Older Population in England: The 2002 English Longitudinal Study of Ageing*, London: Institute of Fiscal Studies.

Marmot, M., Siegrist, J. and Theorell, T. (1999) Health and the psychosocial environment at work, in M. Marmot and R.G. Wilkinson (eds) *Social Determinants of Health*. Oxford: Oxford University Press.

Marmot, M.G. (1997) Early life and adult disorder: research themes, *British Medical Bulletin*, 53(1): 3–9.

Marmot, M.G. and McDowall, M.E. (1986) Mortality decline and widening social inequalities, *The Lancet*, 328: 274–6.

Marshall, G., Swift, A. and Roberts, S. (1997) *Against the Odds? Social Class and Social Justice in Industrial Societies*. Oxford: Clarendon Press.

Martorell, R., Khan, L.K., Hughes, M.L. and Grummer-Strawn, L.M. (2000) Obesity in women in developing countries, *European Journal of Clinical Nutrition*, 54: 247–52.

Marx, K. (1852) *The Eighteenth Brumaire of Louis Napoleon*, trans. S.K. Padover from the German edition of 1869. Moscow: Progress Publishers, 1937.

Marx, K. and Engels, F. (1888) *Manifesto of the Communist Party (English edition)*. Moscow: Progress Publishers, 1952.

Mathers, C.D., Sadana, R., Salomon, J.A., Murray, C.J.L. and Lopez, A.D. (2000) Healthy life expectancy in 191 countries 1999, *The Lancet*, 357: 1685–90.

Mays, V.M., Yancey, A.K., Cochran, S.D., Weber, M. and Fielding, J.E. (2002) Heterogeneity of health disparities among African American, Hispanic and Asian American women: unrecognized influences of sexual orientation, *American Journal of Public Health*, 92(4) 632–9.

McDermott, E. and Graham, H. (2005) Resilient young mothering: social inequalities, late modernity and the 'problem' of 'teenage' motherhood, *Journal of Youth Studies*, 8(1): 59–79.

McKeown, T. (1971) A historical appraisal of the medical task, in G. McLachlan and T. McKeown (eds) *Medical History and Medical Care*. Oxford: Oxford University Press.

McKeown, T. (1979) *The Role of Medicine: Dream, Mirage or Nemesis?* Oxford: Basil Blackwell.

McKinlay, J.B. (1975) A case for refocussing upstream – the political economy of illness, in A.J. Enelow and J.B. Henderson (eds) *Applying Behavioral Science to Cardiovascular Risk*. Washington, DC: American Heart Association.

McMunn, A., Hyde, M., Janevic, M. and Kumari, M. (2003) Health, in M. Marmot, J. Banks, R. Blundell, C. Lessof and J. Nazroo (eds) *Health, Wealth and Lifestyles of the Older Population in England: The 2002 English Longitudinal Study of Ageing*. London: Institute of Fiscal Studies.

Meadows, S. and Dawson, N. (1999) *Teenage Mothers and their Children: Factors Affecting their Health and Development*. London: Department of Health.

Meltzer, H. and Gatwood, R. with Goodman, R. and Ford, T. (2000) *Mental Health of Children and Adolescents in Great Britain*. London: The Stationery Office.

Melzer, D., Gardener, E., Lang, I., McWilliams, B. and Guralnik, J.M. (2006) Measured physical performance, in J. Banks, E. Breeze, C. Lessof and J. Nazroo (eds) *Retirement, Health and Relationships of the Older Population in England: The 2004 English Longitudinal Study of Ageing (Wave 2)*. London: Institute of Fiscal Studies.

Miller, D. (2003) What's left of the welfare state? *Social Philosophy and Policy*, 20: 92–112.

Mills, A., Bennett, S. and Russell, S. (2001) *The Challenge of Health Sector Reform: What Must Governments Do?* Basingstoke: Palgrave.

Ministry of Social Affairs and Health (MSAH) (2001) *Government Resolution on the Health 2015 Public Health Programme*. Helsinki: Ministry of Social Affairs and Health.

Mishel, L., Bernstein, J. and Allegretto, S. (2006) *The State of Working America, 2006–7*. Washington, DC: Economic Policy Unit.

Mitchell, W. and Green, E. (2002) 'I don't know what I'd do without our Mam': motherhood, identity and support networks, *Sociological Review*, 50(1): 1–22.

Modood, T. (2004) Capitals, ethnic identity and educational qualifications, *Cultural Trends*, 13(2): 87–105.

Molarius, A., Seidell, J.C., Sans, S., Tuomilehto, J. and Kuulasmaa, K. (2000) Educational level, relative body weight and changes in their association over 10 years: an international perspective from the WHO Monica Project, *American Journal of Public Health*, 90(8): 1260–8.

Monteiro, C.A., Moura, E.C., Conde, W.L. and Popkin, B.M. (2004) Socio-economic status and obesity in adult populations of developing countries: a review, *Bulletin of the World Health Organization*, 82(12): 940–6.

Morris, L. (1990) *The Workings of the Household*. Cambridge: Polity Press.

Mullard, M. (2004) *The Politics of Globalization and Polarization*. Cheltenham: Edward Elgar.

Mullings, L. and Wali, A. (2001) *Stress and Resilience: The Social Context of Reproduction in Central Harlem*. New York, NY: Kluwer Academic/Plenum.

Murray, C.J.L., Gakidou, E.E. and Frenk, J. (1999) Health inequalities and social group differences: what should we measure? *Bulletin of the World Health Organization*, 77(7): 537–43.

Museum of London, *Bills of Mortality for London for one week, 1665*. www.museumoflondon.org.uk (accessed 17 January 2007).

Najman, J.M. (2001) A general model of the social origins of health and well-being, in R. Eckersley, J. Dixon and B. Douglas (eds) *The Social Origins of Health and Well-being*. Cambridge: Cambridge University Press.

Najman, J.M., Aird, R., Bor, W. *et al.* (2004) The generational transmission of socio-economic inequalities in child cognitive development and emotional health, *Social Science and Medicine*, 58: 1147–58.

National Center for Health Statistics (2001) *Healthy People 2000 Final Review*. Hyattsville, MD: Public Health Service.

Navarro, V. (1976) *Medicine Under Capitalism*. London: Croom Helm.

Nicolaides-Bouman, A., Wald, N., Forey, B. and Lee, P. (1993) *International Smoking Statistics*. Oxford: Oxford University Press.

Norman, P., Boyle, P. and Rees, P. (2005) Selective migration and deprivation: a longitudinal analysis, *Social Science and Medicine*, 60: 2755–71.

Nussbaum, M.C. (2003) Capabilities as fundamental entitlements: Sen and social justice. *Feminist Economics*, 9(2–3): 33–59.

Office for National Statistics (ONS) (2001) *Living in Britain: Results from the 2000–1 General Household Survey*. London: The Stationery Office.

Office for National Statistics (ONS) (2004) *Focus on Inequalities 2004*. London: The Stationery Office.

Office for National Statistics (ONS) (2005) Demographic indicators, *Population Trends*, 122: 6.

Office of Population Censuses and Surveys (OPCS) (1990) *1988 General Household Survey*. London: HMSO.

Office of the Deputy Prime Minister (ODPM) (2004) *Indices of Multiple Deprivation*. London: Office of the Deputy Prime Minister.

Oliver, M. (1996) Defining impairment and disability: issues at stake, in C. Barnes and C. Mercer (eds) *Exploring the Divide: Illness and Disability*. Leeds: Disability Press.

Omran, A.R. (1971) The epidemiologic transition: a theory of the epidemiology of population change, *The Milbank Quarterly*, 83(4): 731–57.

Organization for Economic Co-operation and Development (OECD) (2005) *Society at a Glance 2005*. Paris: OECD.

Palme, J., Bergmark, A., Bäckman, O. *et al.* (2003) A welfare balance sheet for the 1990s, *Scandinavian Journal of Public Health*, suppl, 6: 7–143.

Pampel, F.C. (2005) Patterns of tobacco use in the early epidemic stages: Malawi and Zambia, 2000–2, *American Journal of Public Health*, 95(6): 1009–15.

Pamuk, E.R. (1985) Social class inequality in mortality from 1921–1972 in England and Wales, *Population Studies*, 39: 17–31.

Paull, G. (2006) The impact of children on women's paid work, *Fiscal Studies*, 27(4): 473–512.

Payne, G. and Grew, C. (2005) Unpacking 'class ambivalence': some conceptual and methodological issues in accessing class cultures, *Sociology*, 39(5): 893–910.

Peckham, C.S., Stark, O., Simonte, V. and Wolff, O.H. (1983) Prevalence of obesity in British children born in 1946 and 1958, *British Medical Journal*, 286: 1237–41.

Perry, A., Douglas, G., Murch, M., Bader, K. and Borkowski, M. (2000) *How Parents Cope Financially on Marriage Breakdown*. York: Joseph Rowntree Foundation.

Perry, I.J. and Lumey, L.H. (2004) Fetal growth and development: the role of nutrition and other factors, in D.L. Kuh and Y. Ben-Shlomo (eds) *A Life Course*

*Approach to Chronic Disease Epidemiology*, 2nd edn. Oxford: Oxford University Press.

Peter, F. (2004) Health equity and social justice, in S. Anand, F. Peter and A. Sen (eds) *Public Health, Ethics and Society*. Oxford: Oxford University Press.

Pickett, K.E. and Pearl, M. (2001) Multilevel analyses of neighbourhood socio-economic context and health outcomes: critical review, *Journal of Epidemiology and Community Health*, 55: 111–22.

Pickett, K.E., Luo, Y. and Lauderdale, D.S. (2005) Widening social inequalities in risk for Sudden Infant Death Syndrome, *American Journal of Public Health*, 95(11): 1976–81.

Platt, L. (2005) *Migration and Social Mobility: The Life Chances of Britain's Minority Ethnic Communities*. Bristol: Policy Press.

Pollitt, R.A., Rose, K.M. and Kaufman, J.S. (2005) Evaluating the evidence for models of life course socio-economic factors and cardiovascular outcomes: a systematic review, *British Medical Council Public Health*, 5(7): 1–13.

Population Trends (1993) In brief, *Population Trends*, 72: 1–9.

Powell, M. (1995) The strategy of equality revisited, *Journal of Social Policy*, 24(2): 163–85.

Power, C. and Kuh, D. (2006) Life course development of unequal health, in J. Siegrist and M. Marmot (eds) *Social Inequalities in Health: New Evidence and Policy Implications*. Oxford: Oxford University Press.

Power, C., Atherton, K., Strachan, D.P., *et al.* (2007) Life course influences on health in British adults: effects of socio-economic position in childhood and adulthood, *International Journal of Epidemiology*, in press.

Power, C., Graham, H., Due, P. *et al.* (2005) The contribution of childhood and adult socio-economic position to adult obesity and smoking behaviour: an international comparison, *International Journal of Epidemiology*, 34(2): 335–44.

Power, C., Manor, O. and Matthews, S. (1999) The duration and timing of exposure: effects of socio-economic environment on adult health, *American Journal of Public Health*, 89(7): 1059–66.

Power, C., Manor, O. and Matthews, S. (2003) Child to adult socio-economic conditions and obesity in a national cohort, *International Journal of Obesity Related Metabolic Disorders*, 27(9): 1081–6.

Power, C., Matthews, S. and Manor, O. (1996) Inequalities in self-rated health in the 1958 birth cohort: lifetime social circumstances or social mobility? *British Medical Journal*, 313: 449–53.

Preston, S.H. (1975) The changing relationship between mortality and economic development, *Population Studies*, 29: 231–48.

Preston, S.H., Keyfitz, N. and Schoen, R. (1972) *Causes of Death: Life Tables for National Populations*. London: Seminar Press.

Professional Association of Teachers (PAT) (2002) *Tested to Destruction: A Survey of Stress in Teenagers*. Derby: Professional Association of Teachers.

Qadeer, I. (2000) Health care systems in transition III. India Part 1. The Indian experience, *Journal of Public Health Medicine*, 22(1): 25–32.

Rahkonen, O., Laaksonen, M. and Karvonen, S. (2005). The contribution of lone parenthood and economic difficulties to smoking. *Social Science and Medicine*, 61: 211– 16.

Rawls, J. (1999) *A Theory of Justice*. London: Harvard University Press.

Reay, D. (1998) *Class Work: Mothers' Involvement in Children's Schooling*. London: University College Press.

Reay, D. (2004) Education and cultural capital: the implications of changing trends in education policies, *Cultural Trends*, 13(2): 73–86.

Reay, D. (2005) Beyond consciousness? The psychic landscape of social class, *Sociology*, 39(5): 911–28.

Reddy, S.G. and Pogge, T.W. (2005) *How Not to Count the Poor*. New York, NY: Institute of Social Analysis, Columbia University.

Registrar General (1913) *Registrar General's 74th Annual Report, 1911*. London: Registrar General's Office.

Reid, I. (1977) *Social Class Differences in Britain: A Sourcebook*. London: Open Books.

Rendall, M.S., Joshi, H., Jeungil, O.H. and Verropoulou, G. (2001) Comparing the childrearing lifetimes of Britain's divorce-revolution men and women, *European Journal of Population*, 17(4): 365–87.

Reynolds, T. (2006) Family and community networks in the (re)making of ethnic identity of Caribbean young people in Britain, *Community, Work and Family*, 9(3): 273–90.

Rich-Edwards, J., Kleinman, K., Michels, K.B. *et al.* (2005) Longitudinal study of birth weight and adult body mass index in predicting risk of coronary heart disease and stroke in women, *British Medical Journal*, 330: 1115–21.

Richards, M. and Wadsworth, M.E.J. (2004) Long-term effects of early adversity on cognitive function, *Archives of Disease in Childhood*, 89: 922–7.

Richards, M., Hardy, R., Kuh, D. and Wadsworth, M.E.J. (2002) Birthweight, post-natal growth and cognitive function in a national UK birth cohort, *International Journal of Epidemiology*, 31: 342–8.

Ringdal, K. (2004) Social mobility in Norway, in R. Breen (ed.) *Social Mobility in Europe*. Oxford: Oxford University Press.

Ritakallio, V.-M. (2002) Trends in poverty and income inequality in cross-national comparison, *European Journal of Social Security*, 4(2): 151–77.

Ritakallio, V.-M. and Bradshaw, J. (2006) Family poverty in the European Union, in J. Bradshaw and A. Hatland (eds) *Social Policy, Employment and Family Change in Comparative Perspective*. Cheltenham: Edward Elgar.

Robinson, D. and Reeve, K. (2006) *Neighbourhood Experiences of New Immigration*. Sheffield: Centre for Regional Economic and Social Research, Sheffield Hallam University.

Rose, D. and Pevalin, D.J. (2003) The NS-SEC described, in D. Rose and D.J. Pevalin (eds) *A Researcher's Guide to the National Statistics Socio-economic Classification*. London: Sage.

Rowan, S. (2003) Implications of changes in the United Kingdom social and occupational classifications on infant mortality statistics, *Health Statistics Quarterly*, 17: 33–40.

Royal Commission on the Health of Towns (1845) *First Report of Commissioners of Inquiry into the State of Large Towns and Populous Districts*. London.

Ruspini, E. and Dale, A. (2002) Introduction, in E. Ruspini and A. Dale (eds) *The Gender Dimension of Social Change*. Bristol: Policy Press.

Sacker, A., Clarke, P., Wiggins, R.D. and Bartley, M. (2005) Social dynamics of health inequalities: a growth curve analysis of aging and self-assessed health in the British household panel survey 1991–2001, *Journal of Epidemiology and Community Health*, 59: 495–501.

Sáinz, P. (2006) *Equity in Latin America since the 1990s*, DESA working paper no. 22. New York, NY: United Nations Department of Economic and Social Affairs.

Sameroff, A.J., Seifer, R., Baldwin, A. and Baldwin, C. (1993) Stability of intelligence from pre-school to adolescence: the influence of social and family risk factors, *Child Development*, 64(1): 80–97.

Savage, M. (2000) *Class Analysis and Social Transformation*. Buckingham: Open University Press.

Savage, M., Bagnall, G. and Longhurst, B. (2001) Ordinary, ambivalent and defensive: class identities in the north-west of England, *Sociology*, 35(4): 875–92.

Schooling, M. and Kuh, D. (2002) A life course perspective on women's health behaviour, in D. Kuh and R. Harding (eds) *A Life Course Approach to Women's Health*. Oxford: Oxford University Press.

Schoon, I., Parsons, S. and Sacker, A. (2004) Socio-economic adversity, educational resilience and subsequent levels of adult adaptation, *Journal of Adolescent Research*, 19(4): 383–404.

Secretary of State for Health (1992) *The Health of the Nation*, Cm 1986. London: HMSO.

Secretary of State for Health (1999) *Saving Lives: Our Healthier Nation*, Cm 4386. London: The Stationery Office.

Secretary of State for Health (2004) *Choosing Health: Making Healthy Choices Easier*, Cm 6374. London: The Stationery Office.

Secretary of State for Northern Ireland (1999) *Vision into Practice: The First New TSN Annual Report*. Belfast: New TSN Unit.

Seers, D. (1951) *The Levelling of Incomes since 1938*. Oxford: Basil Blackwell.

Sefton, T. (2002) *Recent Changes in the Distribution of the Social Wage*, CASE paper 62. London: Centre for Analysis of Social Exclusion.

Sen, A. (1984) The living standard, *Oxford Economic Papers*, 6: 74–90. Oxford: Oxford University Press.

Sen, A. (1999) *Development as Freedom*. Oxford: Oxford University Press.

Sen, A. (2004a) Elements of a theory of human rights, *Philosophy and Public Affairs*, 32(4): 315–56.

Sen, A. (2004b) Why health equity? in S. Anand, F. Peter and A. Sen (eds) *Public Health, Ethics and Society*. Oxford: Oxford University Press.

Sen, A. (2004c) Capabilities, lists and public reason: continuing the conversation, *Feminist Economics*, 10(3): 77–80.

Sen, A.K. (1980) Equality of what? in S. McMurrin (ed.) *Tanner Lectures on Human Values*. Cambridge: Cambridge University Press.

Sen, K. and Bonita, R. (2000) Global health status: two steps forward, one step back, *The Lancet*, 356: 577–582.

Sennett, R. and Cobb, J. (1973) *The Hidden Injuries of Class*. New York, NY: Alfred A. Knopf.

Shilling, C. (1993) *The Body and Social Theory*. London: Sage.

Shim, J.K. (2000) Bio-power and racial, class and gender formation in biomedical knowledge production, in J.J. Kronenfeld (ed.) *Research in the Sociology of Health Care*. Stamford, CT: JAI Press.

Shim, J.K. (2002) Understanding the routinized inclusion of race, socio-economic status and sex in epidemiology: the utility of concepts from technoscience studies, *Sociology of Health and Illness*, 24(2): 129–50.

Shonkoff, J.P. and Marshall, P.C. (2000) The biology of developmental vulnerability, in J.P. Shonkoff and S.J. Meisels (eds) *Handbook of Early Childhood Intervention*. Cambridge: Cambridge University Press.

Sigle-Rushton, W. (2005) Young fatherhood and subsequent disadvantage in the United Kingdom, *Journal of Marriage and Family*, 67: 735–53.

Singh, S., Darroch, J.E., Frost, J.J. and the Study Team (2001) Socio-economic disadvantage and adolescent women's sexual and reproductive behaviour: the case of five developed countries, *Family Planning Perspectives*, 33(6): 251–8.

Skeggs, B. (1997) *Formations of Class and Gender: Becoming Respectable*. London: Sage.

Smeeding, T. (2002) *Globalization, Inequality and the Rich Countries of the G-20: Evidence from the Luxembourg Income Study (LIS)*. New York, NY: Maxwell School of Citizenship and Public Affairs, Syracuse University.

Sobal, J. (1999) Food system globalization, eating transformations and nutrition transitions, in R. Grew. (ed.) *Food in Global History*. Boulder, CO: Westview Press.

Sobal, J. and Stunkard, A.J. (1989) Socio-economic status and obesity: a review of the literature, *Psychology Bulletin*, 105(2): 260–75.

Sorensen, G., Gupta, P.C. and Pednekar, M.S. (2005) Social disparities in tobacco use in Mumbai, India: the roles of occupation, education and gender, *American Journal of Public Health*, 95(6): 1003–8.

Sproston, K. and Primatesta, P. (2004) *Health Survey for England 2003, Volume 2 Risk Factors for Cardiovascular Disease*. London: Office for National Statistics.

Stamatakis, E., Primatesta, P., Chinn, S., Rona, R. and Falascheti, E. (2005) Overweight and obesity trends from 1974–2003 in English children: what is the role of socio-economic factors? *Archives of Disease in Childhood*, 90(10): 99–1004.

Steadman, C. (1986) *Landscape for a Good Woman: A Story of Two Lives*. London: Virago.

Studson, M. (1993) *Advertising: The Uneasy Persuasion*. New York, NY: Routledge.

Summerfield, C. and Babb, P. (2004) *Social Trends 34: 2004 edition*. London: Office for National Statistics.

Sustainable Development Networking Programme (SDNP) (2005) *Millennium Development Goals: Bangladesh Progress Report 2005*. Dhaka: Sustainable Development Networking Programme.

Sweeting, H. and West, P. (2001) Social class and smoking at age 15: the effect of different definitions of smoking, *Addiction*, 96: 1357–9.

Szreter, S. (1988) The importance of social intervention in Britain's mortality decline c. 1850–1914, *Social History of Medicine*, 1: 1–37.

Szreter, S. and Mooney, G. (1998) Urbanization, mortality and the standard of living debate: new estimates of expectation of life at birth in nineteenth-century British cities, *Economic History Review*, 1: 84–112.

Tawney, R.H. (1931) *Equality*. London: George Allen and Unwin.

Taylor-Gooby, P. (2005) Is the future American? *Journal of Social Policy*, 34(4): 661–72.

Thankappan, K.R. (2001) Some health implications of globalization in Kerala, India, *Bulletin of the World Health Organization*, 79(9): 892–3.

Thankappan, K.R. and Valiathan, M.S. (1998) Health at low cost, the Kerela model, *The Lancet*, 351: 1274–5.

Therborn, G. (1989) 'Pillarization' and 'popular movements' two variants of welfare state capitalism: the Netherlands and Sweden, in F.G. Castles (ed.) *The Comparative History of Public Policy*. Cambridge: Polity Press.

Thomas, C. (1999) *Female Forms: Experiencing and Understanding Disability*. Buckingham: Open University Press.

Thomson, G.E., Mitchell, F. and Willaims, M.B. (2006) (eds) *Examining the Health Disparities Research Plan of the National Institutes of Health*. Washington, DC: National Academies Press.

Thomson, R. (2000) Dream on: the logic of sexual practice, *Journal of Youth Studies*, 3(4): 407–27.

Thomson, R., Henderson, S. and Holland, J. (2003) Making the most of what you've got? Resources, values and inequalities in women's transitions to adulthood, *Educational Review*, 55(1): 33–46.

Titmuss, R.M. (1943) *Birth, Poverty and Wealth: A Study of Infant Mortality*. London: Hamish Hamilton Medical Books.

Titmuss, R.M. (1958) *Essays on 'the Welfare State'*. London: Unwin University Books.

Townsend, P. and Davidson, N. (eds) (1982) *Inequalities in Health: The Black Report*. Harmondsworth: Penguin.

Tunstall-Pedoe, H., Vanuzzo, D., Hobbs, M. *et al.* (2000) Estimation of the contribution of changes in coronary care to improving survival, event rates and coronary heart disease mortality across the WHO MONICA project populations, *The Lancet*, 355: 688–700.

Turrell, G. and Mathers, C. (2001) Socio-economic inequalities in all-cause and cause-specific mortality in Australia: 1985–7 and 1995–7, *International Journal of Epidemiology*, 30: 231–9.

Turrell, G., Oldenburg, B., McGuffog, I. and Dent, R. (1999) *Socio-economic Determinants of Health: Towards a National Research Program and a Policy and Intervention Agenda*. Canberra: Queensland University of Technology.

United Nations Children's Fund (UNICEF) (2005) *Child Poverty in Rich Countries 2005*, Innocenti report card no. 6. Florence: Innocenti Research Centre.

United Nations Development Programme (UNDP) (2003) *Human Development Report 2003*. New York, NY: UNDP.

United Nations Development Programme (UNDP) (2005) *Human Development Report 2005*. New York, NY: UNDP.

United Nations Economic Commission for Europe (UNECE) (2004) *Thematic Atlas of Europe and North America*. www.unece.org/stats/trends/#ch4 (accessed 20 December 2006).

United States Department of Health and Human Services (USDHHS) Public Health Service (2001) *The Surgeon General's Call to Action to Prevent and Decrease Overweight and Obesity*. Rockville, MD: Office of the Surgeon General.

Variations SubGroup of the Chief Medical Officer's Health of the Nation Working Group (1995) *Variations in Health: What Can the Department of Health and the NHS Do?* London: Department of Health.

Victora, C.G., Vaughan, J.P., Barros, F.C., Silva, A.C. and Tomasi, E. (2000) Explaining trends in inequities: evidence from Brazilian child health studies, *The Lancet*, 356: 1093–8.

Wadsworth, M.E., Butterworth, S.L., Montgomery, S., Ehlin, A. and Bartley, M. (2003) Health, in E. Ferri, J. Bynner and M. Wadsworth (eds) *Changing Britain, Changing Lives*. London: Institute of Education.

Wagstaff, A. (2000) Socio-economic inequalities in child mortality: comparisons across nine developing countries, *Bulletin of the World Health Organization*, 78(1): 19–29.

Wagstaff, A. and van Doorlaer, E. (2000) Equity in health care finance and delivery, in A.J. Culyer and J.P. Newhouse (eds) *Handbook of Health Economics*. Amsterdam: Elsevier.

Wagstaff, A., Paci, P. and van Doorslaer, E. (1991) On the measurement of inequalities in health, *Social Science and Medicine*, 33(5): 545–57.

Wald, N. and Nicolaides-Bouman, A. (1991) *UK Tobacco Statistics*. Oxford: Oxford University Press.

Walling, A. (2005) Families and work, *Labour Market Trends*, 7: 275–83.

Wang, Y. (2001) Cross-national comparison of obesity: the epidemic and the relationship between obesity and socio-economic status, *International Journal of Epidemiology*, 30: 1129–36.

Wanless, D. (2003) *Securing Good Health for the Whole Population: Population Health Trends*. London: HMSO.

Webster, C. (ed.) (2001) *Caring for Health: History and Diversity*. Buckingham: Open University Press.

Wertheimer, A. and McRae, S. (1999) *Family and Household Change in Britain*. Oxford: Centre for Family and Household Research, Oxford Brookes University.

White, C., van Galen, F. and Chow, Y.C. (2003) Trends in social class differences in mortality by cause, 1986–2000, *Health Statistics Quarterly*, 20: 25–37.

Whiteford, P. and Adema, W. (2006) *Combating Child Poverty in OECD Countries: Is Work the Answer?* DELSA/ELSA/WD/SEM(2006)7, OECD Directorate for Employment, Labour and Social Affairs. Paris: OECD.

Whitehead, M. (1990) *The Concepts and Principles of Equity and Health*, discussion paper EUR/ICP/RPD 414. Copenhagen: WHO Regional Office for Europe.

Whitehead, M. (1997) Life and death over the millennium, in F. Drever and M. Whitehead (eds) *Health Inequalities*. London: Office for National Statistics.

Whitehead, M., Dahlgren, D. and Evans, T. (2001) Equity and health sector reforms: can low-income countries escape the medical poverty trap? *The Lancet*, 358: 833–6.

Whitehead, M., Diderichsen, F. and Burström, B. (2000) Researching the impact of public policy on inequalities in health, in H. Graham (ed.) *Understanding Health Inequalities*. Buckingham: Open University Press.

Wilkins, R., Berthelot, J.-M. and Ng, E. (2002) Trends in mortality by neighbourhood income in urban Canada from 1971–96, *Supplement to Health Reports*, 13: 1–28, Statistics Canada Catalogue 82–003.

Wilkinson, R.G. (2005) *The Impact of Inequality: How to Make Sick Societies Healthier*. London: Routledge.

Wilkinson, R.G. and Pickett, K.E. (2006) Income inequality and population health: a review and explanation of the evidence, *Social Science and Medicine*, 62: 1768–84.

Winter, J.M. (1988) Public health and the extension of life expectancy in England and Wales, 1901–60, in M. Keynes, D.A. Coleman and N.H. Dimsdale (eds) *The Political Economy of Health and Welfare*, proceedings of the 1985 Galton Institute conference. London: Macmillan Press.

Women and Equality Unit (2004) *Women and Equality Unit Gender Briefing*. London: Women and Equality Unit, Department of Trade and Industry.

Wong, Y.-L., Garfinkel, I. and McLanahan, S. (1993) Single mother families in eight countries: economic and social policy, *Social Service Review*, 67: 177–97.

World Bank (2003) *World Development Indicators CD-ROM*. Washington, DC: World Bank.

World Bank (2006) *World Development Indicators: Data and Statistics*. Washington, DC: World Bank.

World Bank Development Education Programme (DEP) (2006) *Depweb Glossary.* www.worldbank.org/depweb/english/modules/glossary.html (accessed 19 January 2007).

World Bank website (2006) *Data and Statistics.* http://econ.worldbank.org/WBSITE/ EXTERNAL/EXTDEC/0,,menuPK:476823~pagePK:64165236~piP K:64165141~theSitePK:469372,00.html (accessed 11 December 2006).

World Health Organization (WHO) (1977) *Manual of the International Statistical Classification of Diseases, Injuries and Causes of Death.* Geneva: WHO.

World Health Organization (WHO) (1978) *The Declaration of Alma Ata.* Geneva: WHO.

World Health Organization (WHO) (1981) *Global Strategy of Health For All by the Year 2000.* Geneva: WHO.

World Health Organization (WHO) (1992) *Targets for Health for All.* Copenhagen: WHO Regional Office for Europe.

World Health Organization (WHO) (1998) *Renewal of Health for All.* Geneva: WHO.

World Health Organization (WHO) (2000) *2000 World Health Report.* Geneva: WHO.

World Health Organization (WHO) (2001) *International Classification of Functioning, Disability and Health (ICF).* Geneva: WHO.

World Health Organization (WHO) Task Force on Health System Research Priorities for Equity in Health (2004) *Priorities for Research to Take Forward the Health Equity Policy Agenda* (co-ordinator: P. Östlin). Geneva: WHO.

World Health Organization (WHO) (2005) *Bangkok Charter for Health Promotion in a Globalized World.* Geneva: WHO.

World Health Organization (WHO) Equity Team (2005) *Towards a Conceptual Framework for Analysis and Action on Social Determinants of Health.* Geneva: Commission on Social Determinants of Health, WHO.

World Health Organization (WHO) Europe (1998) *HEALTH21: An Introduction to the Health For All Policy Framework for the WHO European Region.* European Health for All Series no. 5. Copenhagen: WHO Regional Office for Europe.

World Health Organization (WHO) Europe (1999) *Health21: The Health For All Policy Framework for the WHO European Region.* Copenhagen: WHO Regional Office for Europe.

World Health Organization (WHO) Europe (2002) *The European Health Report 2002.* Copenhagen: WHO Regional Office for Europe.

World Health Organization (WHO) Expert Committee (1995) *Physical Status: The Use and Interpretation of Anthropometry.* WHO Technical Report, Geneva: WHO.

Wrigley, E.A., Davies, R., Oeppen, J. and Schofield, R.S. (1997) *English Population History from Family Reconstruction, 1580–1830.* London: Edward Arnold.

Zimmet, P. (2000) Globalization, coca-colonization and the chronic disease epidemic: can the Doomsday scenario be averted? *Journal of Internal Medicine,* 247: 301–10.

# Index

# AN INTRODUCTION TO PUBLIC HEALTH AND EPIDEMIOLOGY
SECOND EDITION

## Susan Carr, Nigel Unwin and Tanja Pless-Mulloli

The contents are not specifically nursing-orientated but very neatly balanced to be of relevance to all working in the public health arena ... the book is well written, the language is clear, and the concepts clearly and simply explained and easily understood

*Journal of Biosocial Science*

- What are epidemiology and public health?
- What is the nature of public health evidence and knowledge?
- What strategies can be used to protect and improve health?

The second edition of this bestselling book provides a multi-professional introduction to the key concepts in public health and epidemiology. It presents a broad, interactive account of contemporary public health, placing an emphasis on developing public health skills and stimulating the reader to think through the issues for themselves.

The new edition features additional material on:

- Historical perspectives
- Public health skills for practice
- Evaluation of public health interventions
- The nature of evidence and public health knowledge
- Translating policy and evidence into practice

*An Introduction to Public Health and Epidemiology* is key reading for students of public health and healthcare professionals, including: nurses, doctors, community development workers and public health workers.

*Contents*
*Introduction – Lessons from the history of public health and epidemiology for the 21st century – Sources and critical use of health information – Measuring the frequency of health problems – Measures of risk – Epidemiological study designs – Weighing up the evidence from epidemiological studies – The determinants of health and disease – Health promotion – Health needs analysis – Principles of screening – Changing public health: What impacts on public health practice?*

July 2007   192pp
ISBN-13: 978 0 335 21624 6 (ISBN-10: 0 335 21624 2) Paperback
ISBN-13: 978 0 335 21625 3 (ISBN-10: 0 335 21625 0) Hardback

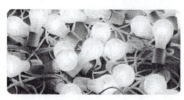
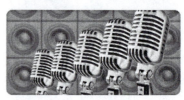
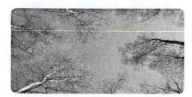
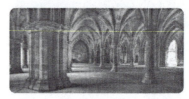
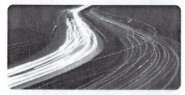
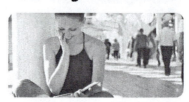
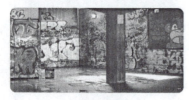